Overview-Map Key

Five-Star Trails

Tucson

Your Guide to the Area's Most Beautiful Hikes

Rob Rachowiecki

MENASHA RIDGE PRESS
menasharidge.com

Five-Star Trails: Tucson

Copyright © 2014 by Rob Rachowiecki
All rights reserved
Published by Menasha Ridge Press
Distributed by Publishers Group West
Printed in the United States of America
First edition, second printing 2016

Editors: Susan Haynes and Tim W. Jackson
Project editor: Ritchey Halphen
Cover design: Scott McGrew
Text design: Annie Long
Cover and interior photos: Rob Rachowiecki except where noted
Cartography and elevation profiles: Rob Rachowiecki and Scott McGrew
Proofreader: Julie Hall Bosché
Indexer: Ann Cassar / Cassar Technical Services

Frontispiece: Rappel Rock from the upper reaches of the *Wilderness of Rock Loop* (*see Hike 16, page 128*)

Library of Congress Cataloging-in-Publication Data

Rachowiecki, Rob, 1954–

Five-star trails, Tucson : your guide to the area's most beautiful hikes / Rob Rachowiecki
    pages cm.

Summary: "Tucson lies in a saguaro-studded desert basin surrounded by four mountain ranges and book-ended by two national parks. In an hour you can drive from an arid canyon in the Arizona–Sonora desert to a pine-forested mountain at 9,000 feet. Hiking trails are plentiful and as varied as the terrain. *Five-Star Trails: Tucson* by Rob Rachowiecki guides hikers to diverse trails suitable for anyone from wheelchair-using nature-lovers to those looking for an all-day workout. Sized to fit in a pocket, this guide is convenient to keep in the car or toss into a backpack. Driving directions steer hikers to the nearest trailhead parking areas, including GPS trailhead coordinates to get them to the start of the trail. Each trail has been thoroughly researched and recently hiked and includes detailed descriptions, trail profiles, and maps. At-a-glance categorical ratings, such as scenery, trail condition, difficulty, solitude, and kid-friendliness, let you quickly select a trail that fits your tastes and ability. Other key information such as fees, restrictions for dogs, and advice on when to visit, offers you the best information so you can plan your trip with ease." —*Provided by publisher.*

ISBN 978-0-89732-442-7 (pbk.) — ISBN 0-89732-442-0
eISBN 978-0-89732-443-4

1. Hiking—Arizona—Tucson Region—Guidebooks. 2. Trails—Arizona—Tucson Region—Guidebooks. 3. Tucson Region (Ariz.)—Guidebooks. I. Title.

GV199.42.A72T8357 2014
917.91'77—dc23

2013045417

 MENASHA RIDGE PRESS
An imprint of AdventureKEEN
2204 First Avenue South, Suite 102
Birmingham, AL 35233
menasharidgepress.com

Disclaimer

This book is meant only as a guide to select trails in and around Tucson, Arizona, and does not guarantee hiker safety in any way—you hike at your own risk. Neither Menasha Ridge Press nor Rob Rachowiecki is liable for property loss or damage, personal injury, or death that may result from accessing or hiking the trails described in this guide. Be especially cautious when walking in potentially hazardous terrains with, for example, steep inclines or drop-offs. Do not attempt to explore terrain that may be beyond your abilities. Please read carefully the introduction to this book, as well as safety information from other sources. Familiarize yourself with current weather reports and maps of the area you plan to visit (in addition to the maps provided in this guidebook). Be cognizant of park regulations, and always follow them. While every effort has been made to ensure the accuracy of the information in this guidebook, land and road conditions, phone numbers and websites, and other information are subject to change.

Contents

Santa Catalina Foothills 135

Saguaro National Park West and Tucson Mountains 177

Madera Canyon Area 217

Dedication

For Audrey Gambach, who shares the trails and trials of life with unflagging optimism, good humor, loving support, and the occasional kick in the pants.

Acknowledgments

Without knowing I was researching a guidebook, many hikers I met provided me with friendly tips and valuable insights. It's remarkable how the whole hiking community looks out for one another on the trails.

I'm equally indebted to the volunteers, rangers, and staff of Saguaro National Park, Coronado National Forest, and Catalina State Park, who likewise were a fine source of information. Again, I rarely revealed my authorship, preferring to receive the same kind of support any other hiker would.

Firefighter David Medford at the Lemmon Rock Lookout cheerfully pointed out some of the highlights of Mount Lemmon. Pima County officials researched my questions about trailheads; in particular, I recognize Regina Nassen and Gregoria Tucker for their service.

I've hiked almost all of these trails more than once, some numerous times. Usually I hike alone, but my daughter Julia joined me on a summit hike of Mount Lemmon, and Audrey Gambach accompanied me at least once on half of these routes. Todd Jones joined us a few times, including on our infamous "pair of drowned rats" hike. (Yes, it *does* rain in the desert.) Thanks, guys!

Lastly, I thank my editors, Susan Haynes, Tim Jackson, and Ritchey Halphen, and my cartographer, Scott McGrew, for putting up with my rants about GPS units—though I still don't know why my parked car was 30 feet lower at the end of my hike than it was when I started.

—*Rob Rachowiecki*

Preface

The highlights of my earliest visits to Tucson in the 1970s were sweeping views of stands of saguaro cactus, those many-armed icons of the desert Southwest. I never took those initial trips in summer, so when the vagaries of life brought me to settle permanently in Tucson in 1989, I discovered that seemingly endless days of 100-degree weather were as much part of the picture as the fabulous desert scenery.

Having been born and raised in England and then having spent a good chunk of my 20s and 30s hiking and climbing in the Andes, I was not very much prepared for blistering summers. Happily, I discovered I could escape into the mountain ranges surrounding Tucson, where lovely forests and temperatures in the 70s provided ideal conditions for enjoying the outdoors.

Perhaps the area's greatest attraction is being able to hike year-round in superb scenery, with gorgeous desert in winter and nearby temperate mountains in summer always providing close-to-perfect weather. Although it is dry in the lowlands, with Tucson averaging a total annual rainfall of barely 12 inches, the mountains form their own microclimates and typically attract two to three times as much rainfall, thus supporting thriving forests.

Mount Lemmon is one of the "sky islands" of southern Arizona. Driving from Tucson to the summit in the Santa Catalina Mountains is the equivalent of driving from the Mexican border to the Canadian border in terms of ecosystems. It takes just an hour to drive Mount Lemmon Road (also known as the Catalina Highway or General Hitchcock Highway) from saguaro cactus lowlands through high desert grasslands and on to oak and mesquite woodlands, ending in pine, fir, and spruce highlands. Meanwhile, the temperature drops by 20°–30°F. It's no wonder, then, that Tucsonans enjoy picnicking and hiking in the mountains to get away from 100°F summer temperatures in the city.

This guidebook includes detailed descriptions of all the best-known routes, ranging from relaxing jaunts of a couple of hours to tough all-day ascents, as well as a number of lesser-known hikes, some of which are rarely described in other books. By no means is this an exhaustive list: Avid hikers are encouraged to discover more possibilities. No overnight backpacking trips are included, although I've suggested a few as extensions or combinations of the day hikes. I've also provided details about campsites that you can use as a base for hiking without having to carry a full pack. But every hike in this book can be accomplished from your home or hotel room in one day or less.

Recommended Hikes

All the hikes in this book are recommended on some level; the following list merely serves as a starting point. There is much overlap among categories, and many hikes could easily fit in several of them. I haven't included a Best for Scenery category—every hike in the Tucson area has great scenery in abundance. Enjoy it!

Best for City Views, Far and Near

Best for Geology

Best for Historical Remnants

Best for Kids

Best for Mountain Summits

Best for Nature

Best for Railroad Views

Best for Ridge Hiking

Best for Seasonal Water Features

Best for Wheelchair Adventurers

Introduction

About This Book

Tucson lies within the Basin and Range Province, a physiographic region that covers much of the western United States and is distinguished by lowland areas alternating with abrupt, high ridges. It's tough country, with vast deserts, precipitous canyons, and steep mountains challenging the original native settlers, early pioneers, and today's travelers.

At an elevation of roughly 2,500 feet, Tucson sits in a basin surrounded by mountains to the north, south, east, and west, some of which rise to more than 9,000 feet and many of which are protected within the Coronado National Forest. In addition, Tucson's fabulous desert scenery earns it two national-park sectors on its doorstep, with Saguaro National Park's east and west districts bookending either end of town. Each district has a visitor center, a scenic driving loop, picnic sites, and numerous desert and mountain trails, but no lodges or drive-in campgrounds.

With more than 500,000 inhabitants and a metro-area population of more than a million, "The Old Pueblo" is a casual city where shorts or jeans and T-shirts or cowboy hats are seen in restaurants, casinos, and theaters. Tucson's cultural quotient is high, however: It's home to the acclaimed University of Arizona; a world-class outdoor museum; thriving arts districts; and more than 20 performing-arts organizations, including both the Arizona Opera and the Arizona Theatre Company. It also consistently ranks atop "best places for bicycling" lists and enjoys 350 days of sunshine a year—perfect for hiking.

The hikes in this book are arranged in roughly doughnut-fashion around The Old Pueblo, beginning on the east side and circling counterclockwise:

SAGUARO NATIONAL PARK EAST AND EASTERN TUCSON The city's east side is bounded by the Rincon Mountains, which rise to more than 8,000 feet. Much of this range lies within Saguaro National Park East, the site of numerous lowland hikes. Two trails that climb into the mountains are described in this book. (The highest peak, 8,666-foot Mica Mountain, is reached by an approximately 26-mile in-and-out hike, not included here.)

SABINO CANYON This is Tucsonans' favorite canyon. Lying at the northeastern end of the city and the southeastern part of the Santa Catalina Mountains, it merits its own recreation-area designation within the Coronado National Forest. The many trails here include some of the best views and most favored water destinations near Tucson. Note that the large parking area can fill early on spring and fall weekends.

MOUNT LEMMON This 9,157-foot peak is the highest in the Santa Catalina Mountains, which abut Tucson's north side and are the city's favored highland-recreation site. The paved 27.6-mile Santa Catalina Highway leaves from Tucson's far northeast side and goes almost to the summit, giving access to numerous hiking trails, picnic areas, campgrounds, a ski area, and the village of Summerhaven. This is the highest road in the Tucson area.

SANTA CATALINA FOOTHILLS Locals simply call this area "The Foothills." Upscale, view-filled housing covers the acreage up to the border with the Coronado National Forest. To the north of this boundary lie some of Tucson's steepest and most difficult trails, climbing beautiful canyons high above the city and into the Pusch Ridge area of the Santa Catalina Mountains.

SAGUARO NATIONAL PARK WEST AND TUCSON MOUNTAINS The city's western horizon comprises the low Tucson Mountains, dominated by Wasson Peak, a panoramic 4,687-foot hiking destination reached by various trail combinations within Saguaro National Park West. My two favorite routes are described in complete detail, and two others are referenced with enough information for hikers to be able to find and follow them to the summit. This range stretches southeast into Tucson Mountain Park, with outlying hills, such as Sentinel Peak, overlooking downtown.

MADERA CANYON AREA The Santa Rita Mountains on the far south side are the highest and most distant from Tucson. The best and easiest way to explore them is to drive to Madera Canyon, which has a wide variety of trails as well as picnic sites and places to stay. Trails vary from wheelchair-accessible routes to ascents of Mount Wrightson, which, at 9,453 feet, is the highest peak in southern Arizona. This canyon also is a favored spot for bird-watchers who come to see the elegant trogon and other species.

How to Use This Guidebook

The following section walks you through this book's organization, making it easy and convenient to plan great hikes.

Overview Map, Map Key, and Map Legend

The overview map on the inside front cover shows the primary trailheads for all 35 hikes. The numbers on the overview map pair with the map key on the facing page. A legend explaining the map symbols used throughout the book appears on the inside back cover.

Trail Maps

In addition to the overview map on the inside cover, a detailed map of each hike's route appears with its profile. On each of these maps, symbols indicate the trailhead, the complete route, significant features, facilities, and topographic landmarks such as creeks, overlooks, and peaks.

To produce the highly accurate maps in this book, I used a handheld GPS unit to gather data while hiking each route, then sent that data to Menasha Ridge Press's expert cartographers. Be aware, though, that your GPS device is no substitute for sound, sensible navigation that takes into account the conditions that you observe while hiking.

Further, despite the high quality of the maps in this guidebook, the publisher and myself strongly recommend that you always carry an additional map, such as the ones noted in each profile opener's "Maps" entry.

Elevation Profile (Diagram)

This graphical element accompanies hikes with significant changes in elevation. Each entry's key information lists the elevation at the trailhead, along with elevations such as the high or low points of the trail, trail ends, or summits.

The elevation profile represents the rises and falls of the trail as viewed from the side, over the complete distance of that trail in miles. On the diagram's vertical axis, or height scale, the number of feet between each tick mark lets you visualize the climb. Varying height scales provide an accurate image of each hike's climbing challenge. For example, the Sentinel Peak hike (see page 196) begins west of downtown Tucson at 2,499 feet, while the Old Baldy and Super Trails (pages 236 and 242, respectively) reach the summit of Mount Wrightson at 9,453 feet, the highest elevation in southern Arizona.

The Hike Profile

Each profile opens with the hike's star ratings, GPS trailhead coordinates, and other key at-a-glance information—from the trail's distance and configuration to contacts for local information. Each profile also includes a map (see "Trail Maps," above). The main text for each profile includes four sections: Overview, Route Details, Nearby Attractions, and Directions (for driving to the trailhead area).

Star Ratings

Each hike in this book was assigned a one- to five-star rating in each of the following categories: scenery, trail condition, suitability for children, level of difficulty, and degree of solitude. This being Tucson, none of these hikes have one- or two-star ratings for scenery—most rate four or five stars. Equally, with trails surrounding a metropolitan area of more than a million inhabitants, it's rare to find a five-star (positively tranquil) rating for solitude. If I can go for an hour without seeing another hiker, I'll rate the hike four stars (spurts of isolation), which is usually as good as it gets. Other categories tend to have more variety among the hikes, but whichever hike you choose, you'll find that it gets four or five stars in at least one and usually two or more ratings groups.

FOR SCENERY:

★ ★ ★ ★ ★	Unique, picturesque panoramas
★ ★ ★ ★	Diverse vistas
★ ★ ★	Pleasant views
★ ★	Unchanging landscape
★	Not selected for scenery

FOR TRAIL CONDITION:

★ ★ ★ ★ ★	Consistently well maintained
★ ★ ★ ★	Stable, with no surprises
★ ★ ★	Average terrain to negotiate
★ ★	Inconsistent, with good and poor areas
★	Rocky, overgrown, or often muddy

FOR CHILDREN:

★ ★ ★ ★ ★	Babes in strollers are welcome
★ ★ ★ ★	Fun for anyone past the toddler stage
★ ★ ★	Good for young hikers with proven stamina
★ ★	Not enjoyable for children
★	Not advisable for children

FOR DIFFICULTY:

★ ★ ★ ★ ★	Grueling
★ ★ ★ ★	Strenuous
★ ★ ★	Moderate: won't beat you up—but you'll know you've been hiking
★ ★	Easy, with patches of moderate
★	Good for a relaxing stroll

FOR SOLITUDE:

★ ★ ★ ★ ★   Positively tranquil

★ ★ ★ ★   Spurts of isolation

★ ★ ★   Moderately secluded

★ ★   Crowded on weekends and holidays

★   Steady stream of individuals and/or groups

GPS TRAILHEAD COORDINATES

As noted in "Trail Maps" (page 3), I used a handheld GPS unit to obtain geographic data and sent the information to the cartographers at Menasha Ridge. In the opener for each hike profile, the coordinates—the intersection of latitude (north) and longitude (west)—will orient you from the trailhead. In some cases, you can drive within viewing distance of a trailhead. Other hiking routes require a short walk to the trailhead from a parking area. (One trail is reached by a motorized shuttle.)

This guidebook expresses GPS coordinates in degree–decimal minute format. The latitude–longitude grid system is likely quite familiar to you, but here's a refresher, pertinent to visualizing the coordinates:

Imaginary lines of latitude—called *parallels* and approximately 69 miles apart from each other—run horizontally around the globe. The equator is established to be 0°, and each parallel is indicated by degrees from the equator: up to 90°N at the North Pole, and down to 90°S at the South Pole.

Imaginary lines of longitude—called *meridians*—run perpendicular to lines of latitude and are likewise indicated by degrees. Starting from 0° at the Prime Meridian in Greenwich, England, they continue to the east and west until they meet 180° later at the International Date Line in the Pacific Ocean. At the equator, longitude lines also are approximately 69 miles apart, but that distance narrows as the meridians converge toward the North and South Poles.

To convert GPS coordinates given in degrees, minutes, and seconds to degrees and decimal minutes, divide the seconds by 60. For more on GPS technology, visit **usgs.gov.**

DISTANCE AND CONFIGURATION

Distance indicates the length of the hike round-trip, from start to finish. If the hike description includes options to shorten or extend the hike, those round-trip distances are also factored here. Where the distances shown on maps and trail signs differ from those I've measured by GPS, I usually favor the former and mention the latter in "Comments" (see next page).

Configuration defines the type of route—for example, an out-and-back (which takes you in and out the same way), a point-to-point (or one-way route), a figure-eight, or a balloon.

HIKING TIME

This book was published as the author celebrated his sixth decade on the planet. Throw in a couple of back and knee surgeries, and I find myself taking 10 hours to hike a trail that was a 6-hour workout a couple of decades ago. Therefore, the hiking times here are geared to my slow pace. Many of you will undoubtedly find my times easy to beat—go for it!

My general rule of thumb for hiking these trails is 1.5 miles per hour, a pace that typically allows time for taking photos, for dawdling and admiring views, and for tackling alternating stretches of hills and descents. Flatter, easier trails can be hiked at 2-plus miles per hour, while some of the steepest, rockiest routes might drop to less than 1.5 miles per hour.

I don't see the point of hiking much faster than 2 or so miles an hour: I prefer to look at the scenery rather than constantly keep my eyes on my feet. I recently hiked off-trail about 10 yards to watch a deer that was munching on a shrub. Several hikers breezed past without noticing me or the deer—their eyes were on the trail. Of course, you don't want to fall, but there is a sweet spot between keeping your eyes *on* the trail and looking *around* the trail.

Finally, when planning to hike a particular trail, consider your general physical condition, experience, expectations, weather, and energy level on a given day.

HIGHLIGHTS

Lists features that draw hikers to the trail: mountain or forest views, water features, historic sites, and the like.

ELEVATION

In each hike's key information, you will see the elevation (in feet) at the trailhead and another figure for the high (or low) point on the trail; where appropriate, a third elevation, such as the trail's end, is also listed. Most hikes also include an elevation diagram (see page 4).

ACCESS

Trail-access hours are also listed here, along with any fees or permits required to hike the trail.

MAPS

Resources for maps, in addition to those in this guidebook, are listed here. As noted earlier, we recommend that you carry more than one map—and that you consult those maps before heading out on the trail in order to resolve any confusion or discrepancy.

FACILITIES

Includes visitor centers, restrooms, water, picnic tables, and other basics at or near the trailhead. In a few cases, facilities may be limited to just a small parking area.

WHEELCHAIR ACCESS

Notes paved sections or other areas where one can safely use a wheelchair.

COMMENTS

Here you'll find assorted nuggets of information, such as whether or not dogs, horses, or mountain bikes are allowed on the trails. I also mention here whether hiking distances listed on maps or signs differ from my GPS measurements.

CONTACTS

Listed here are phone numbers and websites for checking trail conditions and gleaning other day-to-day information.

Overview, Route Details, Nearby Attractions, and Directions

These four elements compose the heart of the hike. "Overview" gives you a quick summary of what to expect on that trail; "Route Details" guides you on the hike, from start to finish; and "Nearby Attractions" suggests appealing adjacent sites, such as restaurants, museums, and other trails (note that not every hike profile has these). "Directions" will get you to the trailhead from a well-known road or highway.

Weather

When Tucson gets rain, it tends to be in the form of scattered showers or focused thunderstorms, and one of the numerous weather stations throughout the city may report twice the daily rain total of another station a few miles away. Tucson's main rainfall occurs during the monsoon season, officially June 15–September 30. Realistically, it rarely rains in June, and the first of numerous monsoon thunderstorms usually falls in the first week of July. These storms can wreak brief havoc on roadways, which rarely see rain and have poor drainage, and some are closed for a few hours. Don't attempt to drive across a closed road. Every year, foolish drivers are swept away by monsoon floods—not all of them survive, and those who do incur hefty fines and rescue fees.

Streams in the lowlands often have water flowing during and after the monsoon, and also in the spring as the snow melts in the highlands. Ski Valley, just above Summerhaven, is the southernmost ski area in the United States; it receives an average of 65 inches of snow in winter. Snowmelt can keep Sabino Creek running into May.

Summer temperatures average 100°F in June and July, but many days are much hotter. Tucson's record high of 117°F was recorded June 26, 1990, and June is considered the area's hottest and driest month. Many Tucsonans escape the heat by driving up nearby Mount Lemmon, but they should be prepared for violent thunderstorms, especially in July and August. Fortunately, these usually occur in the afternoon, making a pleasant hike possible in the morning.

Tucson rarely gets snow, and when it falls it rarely settles, usually melting within minutes. Every few years, conditions might be right to "bury" the city in 2 or 3 inches of snow. Snow-laden branches break, happy schoolchildren get a snow day, and bewildered drivers slide around.

When it comes to avoiding heat, lowland-desert hiking is best from October to April, although nature is somewhat subdued during late fall and into winter. Desert wildflowers are best from late February to mid-April, and depending on winter weather patterns, a spectacular bloom may occur every few years, with golden, white, and blue flowers literally carpeting the ground. Cacti flower reliably from April through early June. Trees noted for their blooms include palo verdes, which are covered in tiny yellow blossoms in April and May. Migrant birds boost avian populations around April, and lizards and other reptiles begin to appear around then.

During the summer, desert hikers need to make very early starts to avoid the heat. "It's a dry heat" is Tucson's summer mantra, and it is true that dry desert air doesn't hold heat as well as moist air does: There is often a temperature difference of 30°F between 4 p.m. and 4 a.m. If pre-dawn wake-ups aren't your thing, drive into the mountains, where flowers bloom well into the summer.

Fall in the mountains brings splashes of color, with the aspens at the bottom of Ski Valley providing one of several reliable shows during the annual Oktoberfest held there. By Thanksgiving, the first snows may have fallen in the high mountains, and it's time to hike in the desert again.

The following charts illustrate the huge variation in climate between Tucson in the lowland deserts and Summerhaven near the summit of Mount Lemmon. For each month, "Hi Temp" shows the average daytime high, "Lo Temp" gives the average nighttime low, and "Rain" lists the average precipitation.

TUCSON INTERNATIONAL AIRPORT

MONTH	HI TEMP	LO TEMP	RAIN
January	66°F	40°F	0.94"
February	69°F	42°F	0.89"
March	74°F	46°F	0.73"
April	82°F	52°F	0.31"
May	92°F	61°F	0.23"
June	100°F	69°F	0.20"
July	100°F	75°F	2.25"
August	97°F	73°F	2.39"
September	95°F	69°F	1.29"
October	85°F	57°F	0.89"
November	74°F	46°F	0.57"
December	65°F	39°F	0.93"

SUMMERHAVEN

MONTH	HI TEMP	LO TEMP	RAIN
January	49°F	23°F	3.15"
February	48°F	22°F	1.69"
March	53°F	26°F	1.17"
April	61°F	32°F	0.50"
May	69°F	37°F	0.25"
June	76°F	44°F	0.62"
July	77°F	50°F	4.41"
August	74°F	50°F	6.99"
September	70°F	45°F	3.39"
October	62°F	36°F	3.05"
November	56°F	30°F	1.75"
December	51°F	24°F	2.60"

A VIEW DOWN PIMA CANYON FROM ABOVE THE SECOND DAM
(see Hike 21, page 158)

Water

A hiker walking steadily in 90-degree heat needs about 10 quarts of fluid per day—that's 2.5 gallons. A good rule of thumb is to hydrate prior to your hike, carry (and drink) 6 ounces of water for every mile you plan to hike, and hydrate again after the hike. On a hot day, you could easily double this amount. In May 2012, two fit young hikers died of heat exhaustion in separate events on popular Tucson trails. The reason: They weren't carrying enough water.

For most people, the pleasures of hiking make carrying water a relatively minor burden, so pack more water than you anticipate needing, even for short hikes. If you don't like drinking tepid water on a hot day, freeze a couple of bottles overnight. It's also a good idea to carry a bottle of sports drink such as Gatorade; the electrolytes replace essential salts that you sweat out.

If you find yourself tempted to drink "found water," proceed with extreme caution. Many ponds and lakes you'll encounter are fairly stagnant, and the water tastes terrible. Drinking such water presents inherent risks for thirsty trekkers. Giardia parasites contaminate many water sources and cause the absolutely awful intestinal ailment giardiasis, which can last for weeks after onset. For more information, visit the Centers for Disease Control and Prevention website: **cdc.gov/parasites/giardia.**

In any case, effective treatment is essential before you use any water source found along the trail. Boiling water for 2–3 minutes is always a safe measure for camping, but day hikers can consider iodine tablets, approved chemical mixes, filtration units rated for giardia, and ultraviolet filtration. Some of these methods (for example, filtration with an added carbon filter) remove bad tastes typical in stagnant water, while others add their own taste. As a precaution, carry a means of water purification in case you've underestimated your consumption needs.

Clothing

Weather, unexpected trail conditions, fatigue, extended hiking duration, and wrong turns can individually or collectively turn a great outing into a very uncomfortable one at best—and a life-threatening one at worst. Thus, proper attire plays a key role in staying comfortable and, sometimes, in staying alive. Some helpful guidelines:

★ Choose silk, wool, or synthetics for maximum comfort in all of your hiking attire—from hats to socks and in between. Cotton is fine if the weather remains dry and stable, not so much if that material gets wet.

★ Always wear a hat, or at least tuck one into your day pack or hitch it to your belt. Hats offer all-weather sun and wind protection as well as warmth if it turns cold.

★ Be ready to layer up or down as the day progresses and the mercury rises or falls. Today's outdoor wear makes layering easy, with such designs as jackets that convert to vests and zip-off or button-up legs.

★ Wear hiking boots paired with good socks to avoid blisters. Flip-flopping along a paved urban greenway is one thing, but you should never hike a trail in open sandals or casual sneakers. Your bones and arches need support, and your skin needs protection from cacti along the trail. Rattlesnakes, while rarely encountered, can't bite through hiking boots.

★ During Tucson's wet months, especially on mountain hikes, don't leave rainwear behind, even if the day dawns clear and sunny. Tuck into your day pack, or tie around your waist, a jacket that is breathable and either water-resistant or waterproof. Investigate different choices at your local outdoors retailer. If you're a frequent hiker, ideally you'll have more than one rainwear weight, material, and style in your closet to protect you in all seasons.

Essential Gear

Today you can buy outdoor vests that have up to 20 pockets shaped and sized to carry everything from toothpicks to binoculars. Or, if you don't aspire to feel like a burro, you can neatly stow all of these items in your day pack or backpack. The following list showcases never-hike-without-them items—in alphabetical order, as all are important:

★ *Extra clothes:* raingear, a change of socks, and depending on the season, a warm hat and gloves.

★ *Extra food:* trail mix, granola bars, or other high-energy snacks.

★ *Flashlight or headlamp* with extra bulb and batteries, for getting back to the trailhead if you take longer than expected (which I often do!).

★ *Hiking poles.* OK, these aren't absolutely essential, but I never hike without them. (European hikers almost always use them.) They take a few miles to get used to, but they help transfer weight from your legs to your shoulders so you can go farther, and they help you balance in tricky spots like creek crossings. Their wrist loops enable you to take a photo or a swig from a bottle without having to ditch the sticks. Try them!

★ *Insect repellent.* Mosquitoes breed during monsoon months.

★ *Maps and a high-quality compass.* Even if you know the terrain from previous hikes, don't leave home without these tools. And, as previously noted, bring maps in addition to those in this guidebook, and consult your maps prior to the hike. If you're GPS-savvy, bring that device, too, but don't rely on it as your sole navigational tool—battery life is limited, after all—and be sure to check its accuracy against that of your maps and compass.

★ *Pocketknife and/or multitool.*

★ *Sun protection:* sunglasses with UV tinting, a sunhat with a wide brim, and sunscreen. Tucson has 350 sunny days per year and ranks second in the world for skin-cancer rates. (Queensland, Australia, is first, if you must know.) Apply sunscreen 30 minutes before you begin hiking, and reapply it after heavy sweating or a dip in a pool or stream. Use a product with an SPF of at least 30, and check the expiration date on top of the tube or bottle. Experienced "desert rats" (as some Tucsonans call themselves) wear light-colored long pants and long-sleeved shirts to protect themselves from the sun, even on the hottest days.

★ *Toilet paper* and a zip-top plastic bag to pack it out in.

★ *Water.* Again, bring more than you think you'll drink. Depending on your destination, you may want to bring a container and iodine or a filter for purifying water in case you run out.

★ *Whistle.* It could become your best friend in an emergency.

★ *Windproof matches and/or a lighter,* for real emergencies—please don't start a forest fire.

First-Aid Kit

In addition to the preceding items, those that follow may seem daunting to carry along for a day hike. But any paramedic will tell you that the products listed here—again, in alphabetical order, because all are important—are just the basics. The reality of hiking is that you can be out for a week of backpacking and acquire only a mosquito bite. Or you can hike for an hour, slip, and suffer a cut or broken bone. Fortunately, the items listed pack into a very small space. You may also purchase convenient prepackaged kits at your pharmacy or online.

★ Adhesive bandages

★ Antibiotic ointment (such as Neosporin)

★ Aspirin, acetaminophen (Tylenol), or ibuprofen (Advil)

★ Athletic tape

★ Blister kit (moleskin or an adhesive variety such as Spenco 2nd Skin)

★ Butterfly-closure bandages

★ Diphenhydramine (Benadryl), in case of allergic reactions

★ Elastic bandages (such as Ace) or joint wraps (such as Spenco)

★ Epinephrine in a prefilled syringe (EpiPen), typically by prescription only, for people known to have severe allergic reactions to hiking mishaps such as bee stings

★ Gauze (one roll and a half-dozen 4-by-4-inch pads)

★ Hydrogen peroxide or iodine

Note: Consider your intended terrain and the number of hikers in your party before you exclude any article listed above. A short stroll may not inspire you to carry a complete kit, but anything beyond that warrants precaution. When hiking alone, you should always be prepared for a medical need. And if you're a twosome or with a group, one or more people in your party should be equipped with first-aid material.

General Safety

The following tips may have the familiar ring of Mom's voice as you take note of them.

★ *Always let someone know where you'll be hiking and how long you expect to be gone.* It's a good idea to give that person a copy of your route, particularly if you're headed into any isolated area. Let him or her know when you return.

★ *Always sign in and out of any trail registers provided.* Don't hesitate to comment on the trail condition if space is provided; that's your opportunity to alert others to any problems you encounter.

★ *Don't count on a mobile phone for your safety.* Reception may be spotty or nonexistent on the trail, even on an urban walk—especially one embraced by towering trees.

★ *Always carry food and water, even for a short hike.* And bring more water than you think you'll need. (We can't emphasize this enough!)

★ *Ask questions.* Public-land employees are on hand to help. It's a lot easier to solicit advice before a problem occurs, and it will help you avoid a mishap away from civilization when it's too late to amend an error.

★ *Stay on designated trails.* Even on the most clearly marked trails, you usually reach a point where you have to stop and consider in which direction to head. If you become disoriented, don't panic. As soon as you think you may be off-track, stop, assess your current direction, and then retrace your steps to the point where you went astray. Using a map, a compass, and this book, and keeping in mind what you've passed thus far, reorient yourself, and trust your judgment on which way to continue. If you become absolutely unsure of how to continue, return to your vehicle the way you came in. Should you become completely lost and have no idea how to find the trailhead, remaining in place along the trail and waiting for help is most often the best option for adults, and always the best option for children.

★ *Always carry a whistle,* another precaution we can't overemphasize. It may become a lifesaver if you get lost or hurt.

★ *Be especially careful when crossing streams.* Whether you're fording the stream or crossing on a log, make every step count. If you have any doubt about maintaining your balance on a log, ford the stream instead: use a trekking pole or stout stick for balance and *face upstream as you cross.* If a stream seems too deep to ford, turn back. Whatever is on the other side isn't worth risking your life for.

★ *Be careful at overlooks.* While these areas may provide spectacular views, they are potentially hazardous. Stay back from the edge of outcrops, and make absolutely sure of your footing—a misstep can mean a nasty and possibly fatal fall.

★ *Standing dead trees and storm-damaged living trees pose a significant hazard to hikers.* These trees may have loose or broken limbs that could fall at any time. While walking beneath trees, and when choosing a spot to rest or enjoy your snack, look up!

★ *Know the symptoms of subnormal body temperature, or hypothermia.* Shivering and forgetfulness are the two most common indicators of this stealthy killer. Hypothermia can occur at any elevation, even in the summer, especially when the hiker is wearing lightweight cotton clothing. If symptoms develop, get to shelter, hot liquids, and dry clothes as soon as possible.

★ *Likewise, know the symptoms of heat exhaustion, or hyperthermia.* Lightheadedness and loss of energy are the first two indicators. If you feel these symptoms, find some shade, drink your water, remove as many layers of clothing as practical, and stay put until you cool down. Marching through heat exhaustion leads to heatstroke—which can be deadly. If you should be sweating and you're not, that's the signature warning sign. Your hike is over at that point: Heatstroke is a life-threatening condition that can cause seizures, convulsions, and eventually death. If you or a companion reaches that point, do whatever you can to cool down, and seek medical attention immediately.

★ *Most importantly, take along your brain.* A cool, calculating mind is the single most important asset on the trail. Think before you act. Watch your step. Plan ahead. Avoiding accidents before they happen is the best way to ensure a rewarding and relaxing hike.

Watchwords for Flora and Fauna

Hikers should remain aware of the following concerns regarding plant life and wildlife, described in alphabetical order. Almost all of these are very rarely seen; if you're interested in a close-up view, visit the outdoor **Arizona-Sonora Desert Museum** (2021 N. Kinney Rd., Tucson; 520-883-2702, **desertmuseum.org**).

AFRICANIZED BEES So-called killer bees are found throughout the Tucson area, though not in abundance. They don't attack unless their hive is threatened, so if you see a colony, stay far away. In rare cases, an attack can be deadly, as happened in May 2013 when a rock climber was found dead on his rope, covered with hundreds of stings.

Most hikers will be able to run away, which is the recommended course of action if you're attacked. Try to cover your face and head as much as possible, don't agitate the bees more by swatting, run into the wind if it's blowing, and move as fast as you can. If you reach shelter, such as your car at the trailhead, get in. (Water is *not* a shelter—the swarm will be waiting when you come up for air.) Bees will follow you for several hundred yards but will give up when you are 0.3–0.5 mile away from their hive. If you get stung, don't try to pluck the stinger out, as this will squeeze the venom deeper into your skin. Instead, scrape it off with your fingernails or a credit card immediately, because the venom sac will continue injecting even after the bee is gone. Get medical attention if you've been stung multiple times or you're allergic to bees.

BLACK BEARS You won't find them inhabiting the desert; however, a small but healthy black-bear population lives in the forests of the high mountain ranges, especially the Santa Ritas. Though bear attacks are uncommon, the sight or approach of a bear can give anyone a start. If you encounter one while hiking, remain calm and avoid running or playing dead. Make loud noises to scare off the bear, and back away slowly.

In primitive and remote areas, assume bears are present; in more-developed sites, check on the current bear situation before your hike. Most encounters are food-related, as bears have an exceptional sense of smell and not particularly discriminating tastes. While this is of greater concern to backpackers and campers, on a day hike you may be planning a lunchtime picnic or munching on an energy bar or other snack from time to time. So remain aware and alert.

CACTI Obviously, you'll see many different species of cactus in prolific numbers. The ones to watch out for are chollas (below), often nicknamed "jumping cactus" because their pads break off and adhere to a passing animal or hiker at the slightest touch. Their spines are barbed and difficult to remove. Carry a comb to pull off the pads

Photo: Fred Gaudet

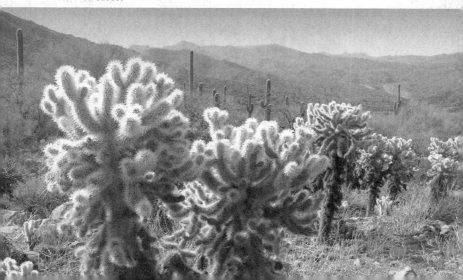

without pricking your fingers. Tweezers on your pocketknife are useful for removing spines.

Also watch out for small pincushion cacti on the ground. They're easy to miss—and no fun to sit on while taking a break.

GILA MONSTERS These are the only venomous lizards in the United States. They are unmistakable, their fat bodies ranging from 12 to more than 20 inches long and covered with beady pink, orange, and black scales arranged in rough stripes. They spend much of their lives in underground burrows, but they come out to feed and mate from April to September, and you might see one on a desert trail if you're lucky. Gila monsters move slowly by lizard standards, and they don't attack. The only way to get bitten is to handle the animal or accidentally reach under a rock where one happens to be resting— very rare and unlikely. When a Gila monster bites, it hangs on to its prey, allowing the poison to sink in, and is difficult to remove. You literally have to pry the jaws off, then get medical attention. The bite can be very painful, but the last recorded death was in 1915.

Photo: Fred Gaudet

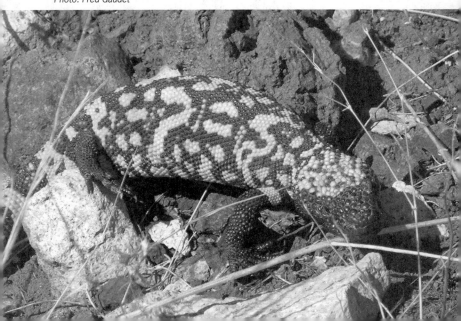

JAVELINAS These pig-like animals live in small herds in the washes surrounding the Tucson suburbs. They've become accustomed to people and their pets, and though they can seem cute and cuddly when young, they have been known to bite. Never feed a javelina (or any other wild animal, for that matter). On trails away from the city, your chances of coming across a herd are low, and the javelinas are likely to run away.

Photo: Doris Evans

MOSQUITOES In some areas, mosquitoes are known to carry West Nile virus, so take extra care to avoid their bites. Pima County, where most of the hikes in this book are located, recorded its first case of the virus in 2003. However, mosquitoes are not especially dense on Tucson trails, even in the monsoon months, so I carry insect repellent but rarely use it until I hear that obnoxious whine.

MOUNTAIN LIONS Also known as pumas or cougars, these big cats are stealthy and rarely seen, but several dozen are estimated to live in the Tucson area. They have occasionally (every year or two) been sighted on popular trails in Sabino Canyon but are more likely to melt into the undergrowth before you see them. If you do encounter one, leave it alone and it will probably go away. If it doesn't, don't run away—it may chase you thinking you're prey. Instead, make yourself as large as possible: Facing the animal, raise your arms and hiking sticks, open your jacket, and pick up small children; speak loudly; and stare the mountain lion down. Remove your sunglasses to make eye contact. Back away slowly while facing the animal. In the unlikely event that you're attacked, fight back with everything you have available: sticks, rocks, packs, swinging camera, bare hands. Keep standing—you're most vulnerable if you crouch.

POISON IVY, OAK, AND SUMAC While you won't find these plants in the desert, they do grow in riparian and forested areas, though not as abundantly as in moister parts of the country. Nevertheless, you need to watch out for them.

Recognizing and avoiding poison ivy, oak, and sumac are the most effective ways to prevent the painful, itchy rashes associated with

Photo: Tom Watson

them. Poison ivy (opposite page) occurs as a vine or ground cover, three leaflets to a leaf; poison oak occurs as either a vine or shrub, also with three leaflets; and poison sumac flourishes in swampland, each leaf having 7–13 leaflets. Urushiol, the oil in the sap of these plants, is responsible for the rash. Within 14 hours of exposure, raised lines and/or blisters will appear on your skin, accompanied by a terrible itch. Try to refrain from scratching, though, because bacteria under your fingernails can cause an infection. Wash and dry the affected area thoroughly, applying calamine lotion to help dry out the rash. If the itching or blistering is severe, seek medical attention. To keep from spreading the misery to someone else, wash not only any exposed parts of your body but also any oil-contaminated clothes, hiking gear, and pets. Long pants and a long-sleeved shirt may offer the best protection.

SCORPIONS Of the estimated 30 species in Arizona, one, the bark scorpion (below), is venomous and potentially lethal. (Only two deaths have been reported in Arizona since 1968.) Light tan in color, this scorpion is barely 1.5 inches long and is most often encountered in woodpiles, under tree bark, or on the undersides of rocks, either near houses or in riparian areas. So don't poke around in fallen wood or pick up rocks or sticks without kicking them over (wearing

Photo: Brian Basgen

a hiking boot) first. A sting from this scorpion is not only dangerous but extremely painful. Fortunately, an antivenin is available, so if you think you've been stung by a bark scorpion, call the national Poison Help Line at 800-222-1222 for advice. The bark scorpion has a slender stinger and pincers; other scorpions tend to be stockier and larger and their bites less painful. Scorpions hibernate from November to March and are most active at night in warm months.

SNAKES In the Tucson region, you will possibly encounter rattlesnakes or corals, which typically hibernate from November to March. Rattlesnakes like to bask in the sun and won't bite unless threatened. Dry scales at the end of their tails produce the well-known rattle—once you've heard that buzzy, low-pitched sound, you won't forget it! If you encounter a rattler, move away from it; the majority of snakebites are caused by people rashly trying to get too close. If you get bitten, loosen tight clothing (including shoes) on the affected limb, remove jewelry, try to raise and immobilize the limb, and get help. Admittedly, this isn't easy to do if you're far from a trailhead, in which case don't attempt to slash and suck—that only makes it worse. Do your best to get to a medical facility, and call 911 or 800-222-1222 for help.

The Arizona coral snake is banded black, white, red, white, and black. The similar-looking but nonvenomous Sonoran mountain king snake (draped over the coral snake in the photo) is banded white, black, red, black, and white. In other words, if the red band is surrounded by black bands, the snake is harmless. In fact, the snakes you'll most likely see while hiking are nonvenomous species. The best rule is to leave all snakes alone, give them a wide berth as you hike past, and make sure any hiking companions (including dogs) do the same.

When hiking, stick to well-used trails, and wear over-the-ankle boots and loose-fitting long pants. Don't step or put your hands beyond your range of detailed visibility, and avoid wandering around in the dark. Step *onto* logs and rocks, never *over* them, and be especially careful when climbing rocks. Avoid walking through dense brush or willow thickets whenever possible.

Photo: Dr. Brendan P. O'Connor

SPIDERS The fearsome black widow, brown recluse, and tarantula can all deliver a nasty bite, but they tend to live in or near buildings rather than on trails. So keep your eyes open when entering restrooms and other facilities near trailheads. If you get bitten, wash the bite with soap and water to prevent infection, and call 800-222-1222 for advice. The spiders you see on trails are most likely benign.

TICKS These arachnids may be found in brush and tall grass, especially during monsoon season. In the Tucson area, ticks rarely attach themselves to humans but frequently bite dogs, so if your pet is scratching, check it for ticks. Remove ticks that are already embedded using tweezers made especially for this purpose. Treat the bite with disinfectant solution.

Hunting

Both districts of Saguaro National Park and the Sabino Canyon area prohibit hunting. Other areas see relatively few hunters. Hunting, often limited to archery, is permitted with a license in some parts of the Coronado National Forest and Tucson Mountain Park during certain short seasons. Some lakes are stocked for anglers with licenses. Contact the Arizona Game and Fish Department for detailed information: 620-942-3000, **azgfd.gov.**

Regulations

Many hikes have information boards at their trailheads informing visitors whether horses, mountain bikes, or dogs are allowed in addition to hikers. Some trails are for hikers only. Where dogs are permitted, they must be leashed. Specific rules are listed in the "Comments" section preceding each hike but are subject to change, so check ahead.

A few trailheads close after dark. This could present a problem if you can't drive out, as in Saguaro National Park East, which is gated at night.

During the dry months preceding the monsoon season, fire restrictions are often enforced. Campfires are prohibited, as are charcoal grills in picnic areas. Hikers wanting to end their trip with a picnic should bring cold food or use a campstove with a shutoff valve. Smoking is limited to cars or buildings with smoking areas. If you hike many of the trails in this book, you'll soon appreciate the damage forest fires have created.

Mountain sheep used to be common in the Santa Catalinas, especially the Pusch Ridge area, but they died out in the 1990s. In November 2013, 30 sheep from the Yuma Mountains, in the southwestern corner of the state, were reintroduced to Pusch Ridge. If this herd does well, more sheep will be introduced, up to a planned total of about 100. Dating from before the new herd, signs at trailheads leading toward Pusch Ridge prohibit dogs and limit humans to developed trails during lambing season.

Other Concerns

Flash floods occur in the monsoon season and can happen with alarming speed. (They aren't called "flash" floods for nothing.) If you're hiking in a canyon area, check the weather forecast and talk to local rangers and volunteers for advice.

Monsoons also bring thunder-and-lightning storms, especially in the afternoon. Try to avoid summits, ridges, and flat, open areas at these times. If lightning is followed by a thunderclap within 5 seconds, the lightning is dangerously close—within a mile or less. To minimize your chances of being struck, crouch down and tuck your head into your hands. Don't stand tall, and don't lie flat. If you're hiking with someone else, keep 20 or 30 yards apart so that you don't both get struck.

Undocumented immigrants and drug smugglers may be encountered near the U.S.–Mexico border. This is generally not an issue in the areas covered by this book, but the Santa Ritas south of Madera Canyon and close to the border are best avoided.

Trail Etiquette

Always treat trails, wildlife, and fellow hikers with respect. Here are some reminders.

★ Plan ahead in order to be self-sufficient at all times. For example, carry necessary supplies for changes in weather or other conditions. A well-planned trip brings satisfaction to you and to others.

★ Hike on open trails only.

★ In seasons or construction areas where road or trail closures may be a possibility, use the websites or phone numbers listed in the "Contacts" section at the beginning of each hike profile to check conditions before you head out. And don't try to circumvent such closures.

★ Don't trespass on private land, and obtain all permits and authorization as required. Leave gates as you found them or as directed by signage.

★ Be courteous to other hikers, bikers, equestrians, and others you encounter on the trails.

★ Never spook wild animals or pets. An unannounced approach, a sudden movement, or a loud noise startles most critters, and a surprised animal can be dangerous to you, to others, and to itself. Give animals plenty of space.

★ Observe the Yield signs around the region's trailheads and backcountry. Typically they advise hikers to yield to horses, and bikers to yield to both horses and hikers. Observing common courtesy on hills, hikers and bikers yield to any uphill traffic. When encountering mounted riders or horse packers, hikers can courteously step off the trail, on the downhill side if possible. So that horses can see and hear you, calmly greet their riders before they reach you, and don't dart behind trees. Also resist the urge to pet horses unless you are invited to do so.

★ Stay on the existing trail, and don't blaze any new trails.

★ Practice **Leave No Trace** principles. Leave the trail in the same shape you found it in, if not better. Visit **lnt.org** for more information.

SYLVESTER SPRING ON KENT SPRING TRAIL (see Hike 30, page 218)

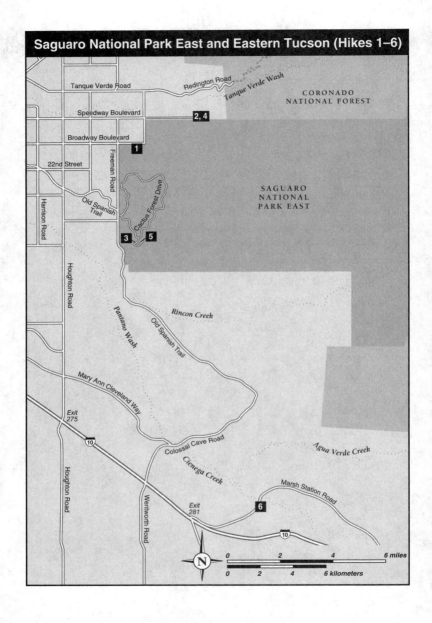

Saguaro National Park East and Eastern Tucson (Hikes 1–6)

Tanque Verde Road

Redington Road

Tanque Verde Wash

CORONADO
NATIONAL FOREST

Speedway Boulevard

2, 4

Broadway Boulevard

1

22nd Street

Freeman Road

Cactus Forest Drive

SAGUARO
NATIONAL
PARK EAST

Harrison Road

Old Spanish Trail

3 **5**

Houghton Road

Pantano Wash

Old Spanish Trail

Rincon Creek

Mary Ann Cleveland Way

Exit 275

Colossal Cave Road

Cienega Creek

Agua Verde Creek

Marsh Station Road

Houghton Road

Wentworth Road

Exit 281

6

10

10

N

| 0 | 2 | 4 | 6 miles |

| 0 | 2 | 4 | 6 kilometers |

Saguaro
National Park East
and Eastern Tucson

UNION PACIFIC TRAINS CROSS CIENEGA CREEK. *(See Hike 6, page 65.)*

Saguaro National Park East:
Cactus Forest–Mica View Loop

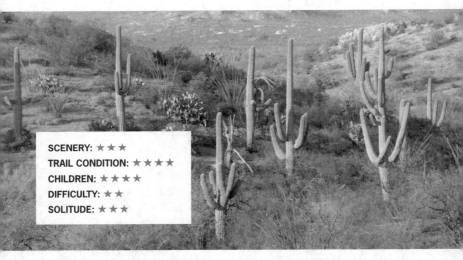

SCENERY: ★ ★ ★
TRAIL CONDITION: ★ ★ ★ ★
CHILDREN: ★ ★ ★ ★
DIFFICULTY: ★ ★
SOLITUDE: ★ ★ ★

SAGUAROS AND OTHER CACTI MIX WITH OCOTILLOS AND MESQUITE TREES ALONG THE TRAIL.

GPS TRAILHEAD COORDINATES: N32° 13.247' W110° 43.570'

DISTANCE AND CONFIGURATION: 10.4-mile out-and-back, 10.5 miles via alternate loop

HIKING TIME: 4.25 hours

HIGHLIGHTS: Varied cactus scenery and views of surrounding mountain ranges

ELEVATION: 2,760' at trailhead, 3,100' at high point

ACCESS: Trailhead open 24/7; park open 7 a.m.–sunset. Admission: $10/$5 per car/pedestrian, payable at the visitor center (4 miles away), valid for 1 week in both Saguaro National Park (SNP) districts; $25 for 1-year car pass. All National Park Service annual passes accepted.

MAPS: National Geographic–Trails Illustrated *237–Saguaro National Park,* Green Trails *Map 2910S–Saguaro;* free trail map available at visitor center

FACILITIES: Parking for about 15 vehicles at Broadway Trailhead; no restrooms or fee station

WHEELCHAIR ACCESS: None

COMMENTS: Horses permitted; mountain bikes permitted on Cactus Forest Loop Drive only; no dogs

CONTACTS: SNP Rincon Mountain District Visitor Center, 520-733-5153/5100, **nps.gov/sagu**

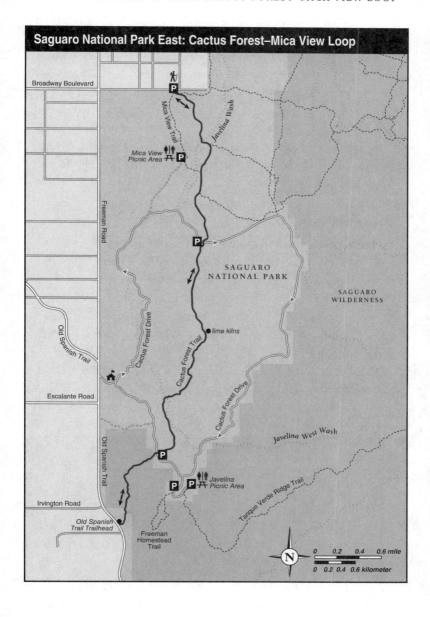

Saguaro National Park East: Cactus Forest–Mica View Loop

Broadway Boulevard

Mica View Trail

Javelina Wash

Mica View
Picnic Area

Freeman Road

SAGUARO
NATIONAL PARK

SAGUARO
WILDERNESS

Cactus Forest Drive

Cactus Forest Trail

lime kilns

Old Spanish Trail

Cactus Forest Drive

Escalante Road

Javelina West Wash

Old Spanish Trail

Javelina
Picnic Area

Tanque Verde Ridge Trail

Irvington Road

Old Spanish
Trail Trailhead

Freeman
Homestead
Trail

N

| 0 | 0.2 | 0.4 | 0.6 mile |

| 0 | 0.2 | 0.4 | 0.6 kilometer |

Overview

This gentle stroll crosses almost the entire girth of Saguaro National Park East from north to south. For a quick look at the desert, you can just take the Mica View Loop (1.9 miles). The northern part of the Cactus Forest Trail intersects several other short trails that can be explored with a map. The main trail intersects the Cactus Forest Loop Drive at two points; mountain bikes are allowed on the 2.6-mile-long section of trail between those points. The remains of late-19th-century lime kilns lie along this section.

Route Details

At the trailhead you'll find a register, map board, and signed trail fork. Take the fork bearing left (south-southeast) and, after 100 yards, take the right fork (southeast) onto the Cactus Forest Trail itself. After about 0.6 mile, you'll cross the sandy Javelina Wash. Surface water rarely flows, but there's enough underground moisture to support a mesquite bosque and numerous low creosote bushes with small, shiny green leaves.

Creosote is a tough desert plant with small yellow flowers that bloom after early-spring rains, followed by cottony white fruits. The plant is nicknamed greasewood because it contains many resins, waxes, and oils that repel insects and grazing animals and give off a distinct pungent fragrance after the first monsoonal rains wash them out. Tucsonans patiently endure the scorching, parched early summer to celebrate that special smell signaling the first cooling rains of late July: "The desert smells like rain!"

A short way past the wash, the Cholla Trail branches left while the Cactus Forest Trail branches right. A few hundred yards farther, the Mica View Trail branches to the right; this can be a short (1.9-mile) loop back to the trailhead or an alternate return from the out-and-back Cactus Forest Trail. Another 0.2 mile takes you to the Mesquite Trail, branching to the left—our trail goes straight on (south) for another 0.6 mile to the paved Cactus Forest Loop Drive. Here, there is parking for five cars if you're visiting by car or mountain bike.

A sign indicates that it's another 0.9 mile south to the lime kilns, to the left of the trail. The foundations on the right side, about halfway to the kilns, are the remains of an early ranger station. At the kilns there isn't much to see, but a notice board provides interesting history and background.

A hundred yards past the kilns, a sign to the left designates a dead-end trail that goes 0.4 mile southeast to Lime Falls, which are dry most of the year. The trail is not very clear, and following it involves crossing a stream several times, but occasional cairns should get you there if you choose.

Cacti, including saguaros, have been plentiful so far, but for a few hundred yards past the Lime Falls turnoff, there are few cacti and almost no saguaros. Soon the trail begins to climb noticeably for the first time on this hike, reaching a ridge with excellent views looking back at the Santa Catalinas. Cross a couple of more ridges, and old-growth saguaros reappear. This is the most scenic part of the trail. Eventually, the trail crosses the unsigned but substantial Javelina West Wash and continues to the second intersection with the paved loop road, 1.5 miles from the lime kilns. Here you'll find

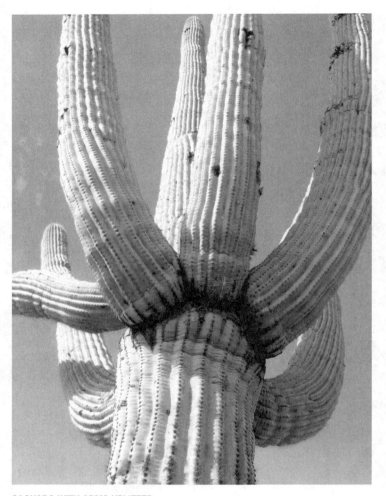

SAGUARO WITH ARMS UPLIFTED

another small parking area for six cars; this is also the end of the trail section where mountain bikes are permitted.

It's 0.9 mile from here to the end of the trail, heading south-west. This is the rockiest and least-maintained part of the trail, and car noise begins to intrude as you approach the final trailhead. To my mind it's the least attractive section, but there is a pretty stand of teddy bear cholla shortly before the end.

Cactus Forest Trail ends at Old Spanish Trail, a fairly busy road—*not* a hiking trail. From this road, the trailhead is unmarked at the time of this writing; there's simply a dirt shoulder on which a handful of cars can park. So if you were thinking of a car shuttle, you just have to know where this dirt shoulder is. If you have a good city map, you can find it on the left side of Old Spanish Trail, 1.5 miles south of the exit of the park and 0.2 mile south of Irvington Road. Good luck with that!

I prefer to make this an out-and-back hike and, when I return to the Mica View Trail turnoff, take Mica View to the left to make an alternate return to the trailhead. This trail passes through the Mica View Picnic Area, which can be reached by car from Cactus Forest Loop Drive. It has a dozen unshaded picnic tables with barbecue grills and a pit toilet, but no water. The area is named for views of Mica Mountain, which at 8,666 feet is the highest point in both the Saguaro National Park and the Rincon Mountains. It's about 12 miles east of the picnic area. From here it's an easy and clear 0.7 mile to the trailhead.

Directions

Drive east on Broadway Boulevard, one of Tucson's longest major east–west thoroughfares. The trailhead and parking area are signed a few hundred yards before the end of Broadway.

From the northwest, take I-10 to Exit 258 and drive 15 miles across Tucson on Broadway Boulevard to the trailhead. From the southeast, take I-10 to Exit 275 and drive north on Houghton Road for 11 miles to Broadway; then turn right (east) and drive 2.8 miles to the trailhead.

2

Saguaro National
Park East: Douglas Spring
and Bridal Wreath Falls Trails

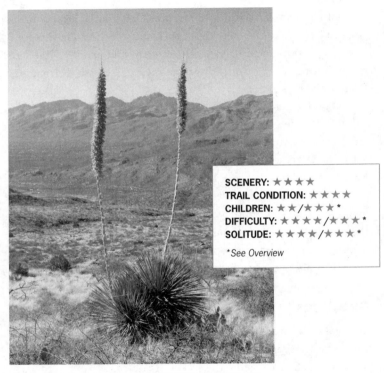

SCENERY: ★ ★ ★
TRAIL CONDITION: ★ ★ ★
CHILDREN: ★ ★ / ★ ★ ★ *
DIFFICULTY: ★ ★ ★ / ★ ★ ★ *
SOLITUDE: ★ ★ ★ / ★ ★ ★ *

*See Overview

**A VIEW OF THE SANTA CATALINA MOUNTAINS NORTH OF
THE TRAIL**

GPS TRAILHEAD COORDINATES: N32° 14.110' W110° 41.215'

DISTANCE AND CONFIGURATION: 13-mile out-and-back to Douglas Spring, 5.8-mile
out-and-back to Bridal Wreath Falls

HIKING TIME: 7.5 hours to Douglas Spring, 3.5 hours to Bridal Wreath Falls

HIGHLIGHTS: Changing scenery, seasonal waterfall

ELEVATION: 2,750' at trailhead, 3,800' at Bridal Wreath Falls, 4,700' at Douglas Spring

ACCESS: Trailhead open 24/7; park open 7 a.m.–sunset. Admission: $10/$5 per

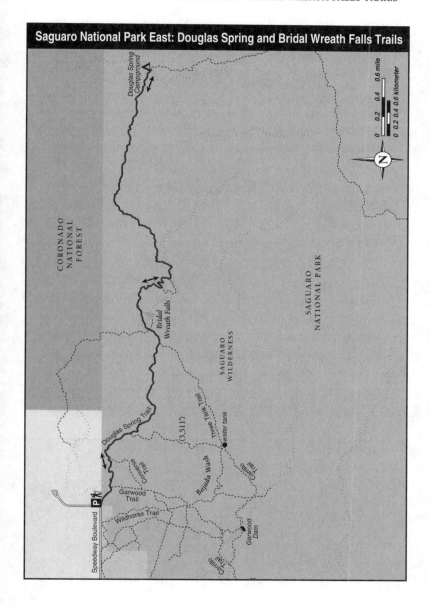

Saguaro National Park East: Douglas Spring and Bridal Wreath Falls Trails car/pedestrian, payable at the visitor center (7 miles away), valid for 1 week in both Saguaro National Park (SNP) districts; $25 for 1-year car pass. All National Park Service annual passes accepted.

MAPS: National Geographic–Trails Illustrated *237–Saguaro National Park,* Green Trails Map *2910S–Saguaro;* free trail map available at visitor center

FACILITIES: Parking for about 20 cars at Douglas Spring Trailhead (horse trailers park at Wildhorse Gate, 200 yards away); shaded benches but no restrooms; no fee station

WHEELCHAIR ACCESS: None

COMMENTS: Horses permitted; no dogs or mountain bikes allowed. Water sources are seasonal and must be treated. Maps and park signs give distances slightly shorter than my GPS measurement.

CONTACTS: SNP Rincon Mountain District Visitor Center, 520-733-5153/5100, **nps.gov/sagu**

Overview

The Douglas Spring Trail is one of two long routes giving access to the west side of the Rincon Mountains from Tucson (the other is the Tanque Verde Ridge Trail; see Hike 5, page 59). Beginning in lowland mesquite forest thick with cacti and ocotillos, the trail soon climbs up small canyons, through open grasslands, and into mid-elevation oak–piñon–juniper woodlands, providing a variety of scenery and birdlife. Many hikers visit the seasonal Bridal Wreath Falls, reached by a short side trail and a good destination for an easier family hike; the second set of star ratings for Children, Difficulty, and Solitude refers to this trip. For an all-day hike, go as far as Douglas Spring, where there is a small backcountry campground (see Nearby Attractions). Hardy, fit hikers can go even farther.

Route Details

From the trailhead, the flat, wide, comfortable trail heads east, passing a trail register after 0.1 mile. Pass a turnoff to your right for the Garwood Dam Loop (see page 52) after 0.2 mile, and then the trail becomes increasingly narrow as it crosses a dry wash and meanders through a mesquite forest. At 0.6 mile, a sign indicates the Converse Trail (shown on some maps as the Wentworth Trail) to your right. Now you start climbing, aided in places by shallow stairs with log or stone risers designed to prevent erosion.

As you climb, glance over your shoulder to your left for fine views of the salmon-colored buildings of the Tanque Verde Guest Ranch below and the Santa Catalinas on the north horizon. The trail swings southeast, briefly follows the right bank of a steep, rocky little canyon, and comes to a junction at mile 1.1, with the Carrillo Trail bearing off to the right (south). Continue southeast to admire a strangely knobby peak on the horizon at 120° southeast—this is Tanque Verde Peak, reached by its namesake trail (see Hike 5).

About 0.5 mile later, the trail flattens briefly, and another landmark appears on the horizon. Helens Dome, a blocky, oblong peak at 80° east, will frequently appear in front of you for the rest of the ascent. You'll drop across a sandy wash that is usually dry and then continue your ascent up the left side of the increasingly steep and rocky drainage, which may have occasional pools of water in it. You'll top out at a point where a pair of aspen trees have decided to spend their lives together, rooted in the middle of the sand, searching deeply for whatever moisture they can find.

The trail flattens and enters an open area of grasses interspersed with cacti, but with few trees or saguaros. In 1989, most of this area was burned by the Chiva Fire, which raged over 9,500 acres high into the Rincon Mountains beyond Douglas Spring. A quarter-century later, it's hard to see where the damage was done.

A sign indicates the turnoff to the Three Tank Trail, on the right at the 2.3-mile mark—our trail continues east and fairly flat for another 0.2 mile to the junction with the Bridal Wreath Falls Trail. The falls trail goes right, slightly south of east, and the Douglas Spring Trail goes left, slightly north of east. (A third trail heads north to the park boundary.)

If you choose the falls, it's barely 0.25 mile to their base, surrounded by a grove of surprisingly large trees that escaped the devastation of the 1989 fire. The waterfall is seasonal and dry most months of the year, barely dripping at other times. If you hit it lucky, after an early-spring snow melt-off or soon after a late-summer monsoon, you could see it in full spate, but this only lasts for several days rather than weeks. Still, it makes a good turnaround point for the shorter hike.

Continuing on the Douglas Springs Trail, you'll cross a stream about 100 yards beyond the junction. If it's running, there's water in the falls. The trail is narrow but clear as it climbs gently through open grassland, with grand views of the Rincons ahead and around and distant vistas of the Tucson valley behind. This section lacks shade and can be tedious on a hot day. Soon, you'll pass through a region of shin-stabbing yuccas, often decorated with impressively tall, flowering spikes that persist throughout the winter.

After a series of switchbacks, you'll notice the flora changing again and becoming bushier, with small trees. On the right, a shallow, rocky watercourse may have pools of water or even a trickling stream. The variety of vegetation and splashes of water attract wildlife. When I hiked in March, I met an excited young woman who told me that she had just seen her first mountain lion. All I saw were a pair of deer, some squirrels, and a variety of birds. By April, you should keep your eyes open for lizards and especially rattlesnakes.

For the final almost 2 miles, the trail undulates, cresting false ridges and dropping down, occasionally crossing a damp spot if there

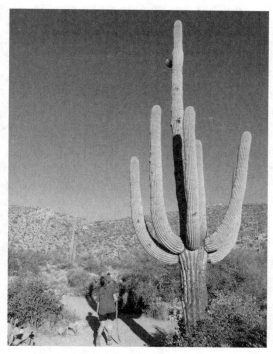

**JUNCTION OF THE DOUGLAS SPRING AND
CARRILLO TRAILS**

has been rain, until finally it reaches the high point, a few hundred
yards before reaching Douglas Spring Campground. A sign indicates
an elevation of 4,800 feet, but it's about 100 feet lower on most topographic maps. Water is available for several months of the year from
the spring, which is on the right of the trail just before the campground, but it shouldn't be relied on and needs to be treated. There
are a handful of campsites and an ugly vault toilet—reportedly it was
far prettier before the 1989 fire.

Tough, fit hikers can continue south on the Douglas Spring
Trail for about 2.4 miles to Cow Head Saddle at about 6,150 feet,
and beyond. With a car shuttle, you could take the Tanque Verde
Ridge Trail (see page 59) from Cow Head another 11.6 miles—this is

a 20.5-mile all-day hike that I did once, 30 years ago. Most hikers will turn around and retrace their footsteps to the trailhead.

Nearby Attractions

Though this book is a guide for day hikers, it's worth noting that some of Tucson's best backcountry backpacking is found in Saguaro National Park's Rincon Mountain (East) District. The entire park has only six small backcountry-camping areas, all in this district. Douglas Spring is the closest to a parking area and gives access to trails crossing the high Rincon peaks. A permit is necessary, available from the visitor center for $6 per night, per site. Rangers are on hand to discuss recent reports on the availability of water and possible onward routes into the high Rincons. No campfires are allowed here.

For more information about the visitor center, see the next hike.

Directions

Drive east on Speedway Boulevard, Tucson's longest major east–west thoroughfare. Continue until Speedway dead-ends, and turn right into the parking area for the Douglas Spring Trailhead.

From Saguaro National Park's eastern visitor center, drive west 0.1 mile to Old Spanish Trail, turn right, and drive north 0.1 mile. Where Old Spanish Trail veers left (northwest), continue north on the minor Freeman Road for 3.6 miles to Speedway Boulevard; then turn right (east) on Speedway and drive 3 miles to the trailhead.

From the northwest, take I-10 to Exit 257 and cross Tucson on Speedway Boulevard for 17.5 miles to the trailhead. From the southeast, take I-10 to Exit 275 and drive north on Houghton Road for 12 miles; then turn right (east) on Speedway and drive 5 miles to the trailhead.

3

Saguaro National Park
East: Freeman Homestead Trail

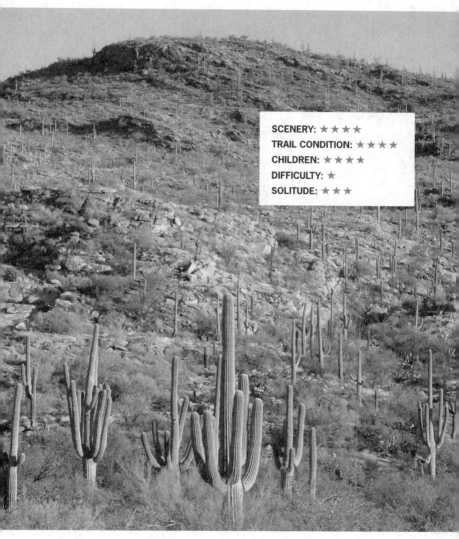

SCENERY: ★ ★ ★
TRAIL CONDITION: ★ ★ ★
CHILDREN: ★ ★ ★
DIFFICULTY: ★
SOLITUDE: ★ ★

STANDS OF MATURE SAGUAROS ARE ESPECIALLY THICK HERE.

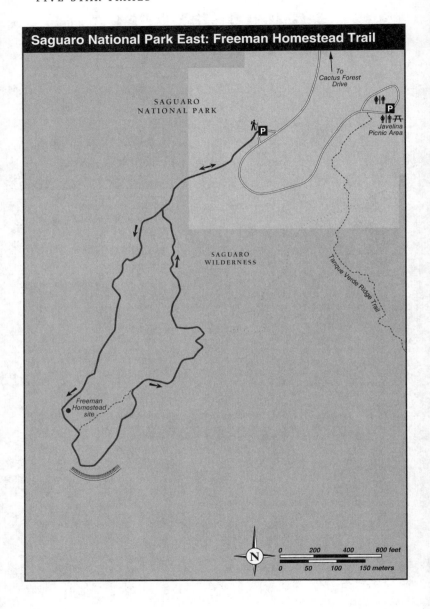

Saguaro National Park East: Freeman Homestead Trail

GPS TRAILHEAD COORDINATES: N32° 09.916' W110° 43.561'

DISTANCE AND CONFIGURATION: 1.1-mile balloon

HIKING TIME: 1 hour

HIGHLIGHTS: Exploratory nature and history trail; saguaros galore

ELEVATION: 3,105' at trailhead, 2,919' at low point

ACCESS: Open 7 a.m.–sunset. Admission: $10/$5 per car/pedestrian, payable at the visitor center (almost 2 miles away), valid for 1 week in both Saguaro National Park districts; $25 for 1-year car pass. All National Park Service annual passes accepted.

MAPS: National Geographic–Trails Illustrated *237–Saguaro National Park*, Green Trails Map *2910S–Saguaro;* free trail map available at visitor center

FACILITIES: Visitor center (see Nearby Attractions); Javelina Picnic Area (with pit toilets and parking) 0.3 mile away; parking at trailhead for 6 cars; no water

WHEELCHAIR ACCESS: None

COMMENTS: No pets, horses, or mountain bikes allowed. Don't return after sunset— the gates close soon after and you can't drive out.

CONTACTS: SNP Rincon Mountain District Visitor Center, 520-733-5153/5100, nps.gov/sagu

Overview

This is a fun loop for families, with several interpretive stations providing information about the desert for adults, as well as kid-oriented questions or puzzles for the younger members of your group. The stands of saguaros are especially thick and impressive in this area. There are steps and sandy spots in a few places, so strollers aren't recommended. Sure, you could lope around the trail in 20 minutes, but it's worth taking the time and enjoying this introduction to the national park.

Route Details

The trail gets its name from Safford and Viola Freeman, who applied to homestead 640 acres in the area in 1929 and built a three-room adobe house here in 1930, with outbuildings housing a separate kitchen and storage areas. They built an access road that later became Old Spanish Trail, which you probably drove to reach Saguaro National Park. The family lived on the property until 1934, the year after Saguaro National Monument was established. After they left to return to Tucson, Safford Freeman's father continued to homestead here. The family sold the house and land to the federal government in 1951, and the acreage became part of the national monument. Apart from remnants of some foundations, nothing is left of the Freeman family's home except an open space in the desert vegetation.

If you can't find a spot in the six-car parking area at the trailhead, you can park at the nearby Javelina Picnic Area and walk back along the road. From the trailhead, the path goes southwest; formed of loose sand and small rocks, it descends imperceptibly through creosote, Mormon tea, prickly pear, and other plants. Just over 0.1 mile along the trail, you reach a fork. Signs indicate that you should take the right fork, taking the loop counterclockwise. This will help you meet and read interpretive trail signs more easily.

As you descend, occasionally down simple steps, you'll see ever more saguaros. Some of them are huge, up to 50 feet in height and carrying 15 or 20 arms. Reportedly, there's a 30-arm saguaro here, but I haven't found it. These mature cacti might exceed 150 years in age, and most of their growing is done in the latter half of their lives. It can take 15 years for seedlings to reach more than a foot in height, and 75 years before they first start growing their distinctive arms. Nevertheless, they can flower and fruit while still quite young, and a 4-foot-tall, 30-year-old saguaro may boast its first distinctive crown of white flowers in May, followed by red fruits in June.

When you reach the homestead site, you'll find a couple of benches where you can sit down, take in the views, and consider what life must have been like here more than 80 years ago. The homestead itself was behind the benches, and parts of the concrete floor slab remain. A berm near the foundation suggests that a fence once stood here, supposedly made of ocotillo branches.

After you finish looking over the area, continue by skirting widely to the right (west) side of the site and finding the trail, which continues south and reaches a wash and cliff about 0.1 mile south of the homestead. Here, turn sharply left and follow the wash as it swings east and northeast. There isn't much of a trail here—you simply follow the bottom of the wash, aided by an occasional concrete slab etched with an arrow. About 0.3 mile along the wash, which, fortunately, is almost always dry, look for the trail breaking away to the north from the left bank.

The trail climbs north for a few hundred yards and reaches the fork that you took near the beginning of the hike. Turn right here to return to the trailhead.

Nearby Attractions

The **Rincon Mountain District Visitor Center** of Saguaro National Park (upgraded from a national monument in 1994) is also the park head- quarters. At the park entrance, at 3693 Old Spanish Trail, it's open daily, 9 a.m.–5 p.m., except December 25. Inside you'll find restrooms, a gift shop, exhibits, and rangers on duty who can provide maps, information, and backcountry-camping permits. No food or drink is sold, but water is available so you can fill your own bottle.

Continuing into the park, the 8-mile, one-way **Cactus Forest Drive**—the only road in the eastern sector of the park—provides

PRICKLY PEAR CACTI AND A GHOST SAGUARO GUARD THE TRAIL.

excellent views and access to various overlooks and trails. If you haven't been here before, you should certainly experience it before going to the Freeman Homestead Trail.

Directions

From central Tucson, take 22nd Street east to Old Spanish Trail, which is 0.2 mile east of Harrison Road. Bear right onto Old Spanish Trail, following it southeast for 4 miles to the park entrance and visitor center. Shortly past the visitor center, Cactus Forest Drive forks—take the right fork 1.2 miles to the trailhead.

Coming from the northwest, take 1-10 to Exit 259, drive east on 22nd Street for 11.3 miles to Old Spanish Trail, and continue as described above. Coming from the southeast, take I-10 to Exit 275 and drive north on Houghton Road for 8 miles to Escalante Road. Turn right (east) on Escalante and drive 2 miles to Old Spanish Trail, where you turn left and drive north 0.3 mile to the park entrance.

Saguaro National Park
East: Garwood Dam Loop

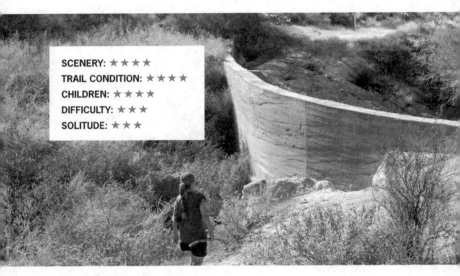

SCENERY: ★ ★ ★ ★
TRAIL CONDITION: ★ ★ ★ ★
CHILDREN: ★ ★ ★ ★
DIFFICULTY: ★ ★ ★
SOLITUDE: ★ ★ ★

EXPLORING GARWOOD DAM

GPS TRAILHEAD COORDINATES: N32° 14.110' W110° 41.215'

DISTANCE AND CONFIGURATION: 5.6-mile loop

HIKING TIME: 3 hours

HIGHLIGHTS: Superb saguaro forest, historical dam

ELEVATION: 2,750' at trailhead, 3,511' on Carrillo Trail

ACCESS: Trailhead open 24/7; park open 7 a.m.–sunset. Admission: $10/$5 per car/
pedestrian, payable at the visitor center (7 miles away), valid for 1 week in both
Saguaro National Park districts; $25 for 1-year car pass. All National Park Service
annual passes accepted.

MAPS: National Geographic–Trails Illustrated 237–Saguaro National Park, Green Trails Map
2910S–Saguaro; free trail map available at visitor center

FACILITIES: Parking for about 20 cars at Douglas Spring Trailhead (horse trailers park at
Wildhorse Gate, 200 yards away); shaded benches but no restrooms; no fee station

WHEELCHAIR ACCESS: None

COMMENTS: Horses permitted; no dogs or mountain bikes allowed. Maps and park signs
show distances slightly shorter than my GPS measurement.

CONTACTS: SNP Rincon Mountain District Visitor Center, 520-733-5153/5100,
nps.gov/sagu

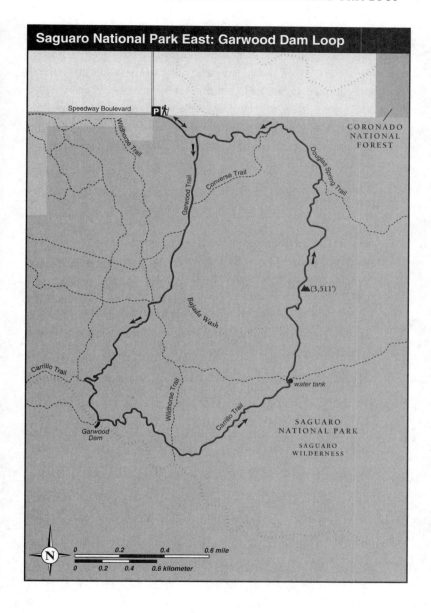

Overview

This enjoyable loop is one of dozens that can be put together from the dense network of trails lacing the northwestern corner of the national park. Unlike most of the other loops, this one provides 760 feet of elevation gain, allowing much better views than the lower trails immediately to the west. The thick saguaro forest includes the rare cristate form of the cactus, and a small dam and water tank provide insights into Tucson's history three-quarters of a century ago.

Route Details

From the trailhead, the flat, wide, comfortable Douglas Spring Trail (see page 38) heads east, passing a trail register after 0.1 mile. When you reach the signed Garwood Trail junction, after 0.2 mile, turn right (south) onto a sandy, narrow trail. The sand is compacted at just the right consistency—hard enough to walk on without slipping, yet soft enough to provide cushioning for your feet. Perfect!

The surroundings are lush by desert standards, with mesquite trees, creosote bushes, ocotillos, and many different cacti providing cover for wildlife. This is a wonderful place to hike during the first rains of the monsoon, when the pungent perfumes of the summer-dried plants are released.

Looking straight ahead (south), you'll admire the views of Tanque Verde Ridge that dominate the horizon. Almost 0.5 mile along, a metal sign marks the Converse Trail, which for some puzzling reason is marked as Wentworth Trail on most maps. Continue south on the Garwood Trail for 0.4 mile farther, crossing the signed and usually dry Bajada Wash, and in another 0.1 mile you come to a junction where six trails converge.

Here there are three signs, so check them all to make sure you continue on the Garwood Trail, which soon swings around to the southwest. After 0.4 mile, cross another dry wash, this one remarkable for the cristate saguaro growing next to it. Soon the trail follows a couple of gentle switchbacks, taking you to a minor ridge where you intersect the Carrillo Trail, named after Emilio Carrillo, who built his Buena Vista Ranch in 1868 on what later became the Tanque Verde Guest Ranch (see Nearby Attractions). Take this trail to the left, going briefly east and then swinging south and southeast and climbing around the back of the minor ridge.

About 0.3 mile along the Carrillo Trail, you'll reach the substantial Garwood Dam on your right. It was built by Nelson Garwood, who bought 480 acres in the area in 1945. To reach the property, he constructed a rudimentary road by dragging railroad ties behind his jeep along what is now the Garwood Trail, though it's hard to see signs of that today. In 1948 he began building the dam and a ranch house, although he never introduced cattle onto his property. The dam was intended to supply permanent water for the house, and he lived there with his family for some years while selling segments of his property. In 1959 he sold everything, and the house stood empty for years. Vandals burned it in the early 1970s, and the National Park Service took over the property soon after.

There may be pools of water behind the dam, and you'll enjoy good views from here of the Tucson valley and the Tucson Mountains beyond. It's a good spot for wildflowers in spring, and the smooth rocks behind the dam invite you to sit and have a snack. While the dam looks sturdy, it's dangerous to walk across.

THE TOP OF A CRISTATE SAGUARO

Continue climbing generally east from the dam along the Carrillo Trail, passing the intersection with the north and south arms of the Wildhorse Trail, 0.6 mile away, and continuing up to a round steel tank, 0.8 mile beyond the intersection. Several tanks are marked on park maps. Originally, most of these were natural rock pools that were deep and shaded enough to hold water year-round; they were also important places for the original Native American inhabitants and later for cattle ranchers who used to lease these lands. Today they are of historical interest—the last grazing lease in the park expired in 1979.

The steel tank is unusual in that it's not a natural formation: It was constructed to hold water from nearby Rock Spring. About 8 feet high and 20 feet across, it's quite an impressive structure, albeit no longer in use. Tanks would often get stagnant and covered with green algae, hence the ubiquitous name Tanque Verde, Spanish for "green tank." To solve the algae problem, ranchers used to stock the tanks with goldfish to eat the algae.

Four trails converge at the tank, which you need to walk around and behind to find the continuation of the Carrillo Trail, now climbing north. Ahead of you is a gently sloping pyramidal peak, marked simply as 3,511 on topographic maps. This will be the highest point of our loop, 0.5 mile north of the tank.

From the summit, enjoy great views of the Santa Catalinas to the north, the Rincons to the east, Tanque Verde Ridge to the south, and the Tucson valley to the east. You can even pick out your car waiting in the parking lot just over a mile away to the northwest.

Carrillo Trail now descends quite steeply north and, after several hundred yards, flattens and follows a narrow gully that might require wading after heavy rains. The route goes west briefly before swinging north again and reaching a huge saguaro—this marks the intersection with the Douglas Spring Trail, which takes you to the parking area, 0.6 mile away. Turn left (northwest) and descend along the north side of a hill with expansive views of the Santa Catalinas and Tanque Verde Guest Ranch. In places the route has been stabilized with wide steps formed with log or stone risers. Soon you'll pass the turnoff to the left for the Converse Trail, cross a sandy wash, and continue past the beginning of the Garwood Trail and on to the parking area.

Nearby Attractions

Tanque Verde Guest Ranch is a high-end dude ranch immediately north of the parking area. With 75 rooms and 180 horses, there's a perfect mount for everyone. While guided horseback riding, sometimes into the national park, is the main focus, the ranch also prides itself on its comfortable rooms and suites, fine dining, and barbecue meals served at the end of a trail ride, sometimes with old-fashioned Western entertainment. Riding lessons are available, as are children's programs. Mountain biking, fishing, and hiking are offered; guests can also use indoor and outdoor pools, a nature center, and a tennis court, as well as avail themselves of spa, yoga, fitness, wellness, and arts-and-crafts programs.

At press time, all-inclusive rates run $480–$800 per night (double occupancy); prices include tax and are dependent on season and room. More-expensive haciendas with private patios are also available. More information: 800-234-3833, **tanqueverderanch.com.**

Directions

Drive east on Speedway Boulevard, Tucson's longest major east–west thoroughfare. Continue until Speedway dead-ends, and turn right into the parking area for the Douglas Spring Trailhead.

From Saguaro National Park's eastern visitor center, drive west 0.1 mile to Old Spanish Trail, turn right, and drive north 0.1 mile. Where Old Spanish Trail veers left (northwest), continue north on the minor Freeman Road for 3.6 miles to Speedway Boulevard; then turn right (east) on Speedway and drive 3 miles to the trailhead.

From the northwest, take I-10 to Exit 257 and cross Tucson on Speedway Boulevard for 17.5 miles to the trailhead. From the southeast, take I-10 to Exit 275 and drive north on Houghton Road for 12 miles to Speedway Boulevard; then turn right (east) on Speedway and drive 5 miles to the trailhead.

5

Saguaro National Park
East: Tanque Verde Ridge Trail

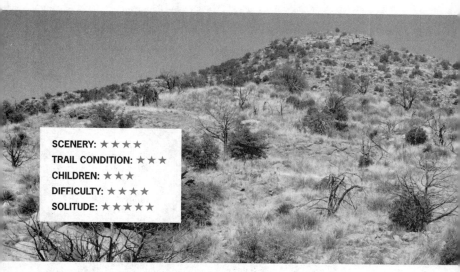

SCENERY: ★ ★ ★ ★
TRAIL CONDITION: ★ ★ ★
CHILDREN: ★ ★ ★
DIFFICULTY: ★ ★ ★ ★
SOLITUDE: ★ ★ ★ ★ ★

YUCCAS ON THE MID-LEVELS OF THE TANQUE VERDE RIDGE TRAIL

GPS TRAILHEAD COORDINATES: N32° 09.938' W110° 43.437'

DISTANCE AND CONFIGURATION: 13.8-mile out-and-back

HIKING TIME: 9 hours

HIGHLIGHTS: Views of the Tucson Basin surrounded by the Santa Catalina, Tucson, and Santa Rita Mountains; vegetation changes

ELEVATION: 3,115' at trailhead, 5,983' at Juniper Basin campsite

ACCESS: Open 7 a.m.–sunset. Admission: $10/$5 entrance per car/pedestrian, payable at the visitor center (1.6 miles away), valid for 1 week in both districts; $25 for 1-year car pass; all National Park Service annual passes accepted.

MAPS: National Geographic–Trails Illustrated *237–Saguaro National Park*, Green Trails *Map 2910S–Saguaro*; free trail map available at visitor center

FACILITIES: Javelina Picnic Area (with pit toilets and parking) at trailhead; no water; visitor center

WHEELCHAIR ACCESS: None except for the Javelina Picnic Area

COMMENTS: Hikers only. Don't return after sunset—the gates close soon after and you can't drive out.

CONTACTS: SNP Rincon Mountain District Visitor Center, 520-733-5153/5100, **nps.gov/sagu**

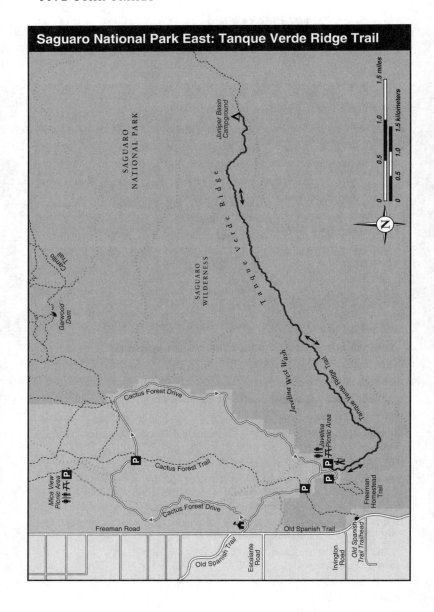

Saguaro National Park East: Tanque Verde Ridge Trail

Overview

Tanque Verde Ridge is the westernmost mountain finger pointing toward Tucson from the Rincons. As you climb it, views of all the other ranges surrounding the city open, and on clear days you can see into Mexico as well as many of the other minor ranges in southern Arizona. Starting in lush desert vegetation, you'll climb through grasslands and into piñon–juniper vegetation to the small Juniper Basin campsite.

Route Details

The trailhead is on the right side of the entrance of the Javelina Picnic Area, clearly marked with an information board and map. Looking south from the picnic area, you can see Tanque Verde Ridge, up which you'll be hiking, on the horizon.

The flat, narrow trail heads southwest through thick desert vegetation of cacti and ocotillos. During your first 5 minutes of hiking you'll swing southeast, drop and cross a small wash that's usually dry, and reach a trail register where you're encouraged to sign in.

This is the last signpost until you reach the Juniper Basin campsite, almost 7 miles up the ridge.

The trail now climbs southeast toward Tanque Verde Ridge. A few false trails break off to the right, affording better views of Tucson, but keep climbing and dipping a couple of times through almost imperceptible dry stream beds. Views of the Tucson basin will open up. Looking a few miles due west, you'll see an open area dotted with rows of tiny ... *what*? With binoculars, you can make out that these are aircraft, wrapped and stored in what locals call "The Boneyard." There are more than 4,000 military planes here, of no use at the present but which might fly or be used for parts in the future. See Nearby Attractions for more details.

As you climb toward 4,000 feet elevation, you'll pass through thick stands of ocotillo (*Fouquieria splendens*), one of my favorite desert plants. For much of the year they look like bare, dead, thorny sticks reaching 20 feet tall, but after rains they sprout short-lived small green leaves along the stems. In dry months, the leaves are shed and the cycle can repeat itself during the year. Ocotillos have bright-red clusters of sweet tubular flowers at the tips of the sticks from March through early summer, swaying colorfully in spring breezes and attracting hummingbirds, orioles, and carpenter bees. Traditionally, the stems have been planted to make impenetrable fences and sometimes have been used as support for mud-daubed walls and shade ramadas. Some of the largest plants can live as long as 100 years.

Just over a mile into the hike, after climbing steadily, the clear trail flattens out for about 100 yards and then climbs through a few rock slabs where the path is not obvious—look for cairns to guide you through the bare spots. As you climb the ridge, you'll find many more sections where you'll need to keep your eyes open for cairns. Meanwhile, you can now admire the views of the Catalinas to the north and the Santa Ritas to the south. Southern Arizona's highest peak, Mount Wrightson, is the uppermost point, roughly in the middle of the Santa Ritas, and if you follow the view of the range to the right, the westernmost peak is Elephant Head. With a tiny dose of imagination, you can see how that peak got its name.

At around 4,300 feet elevation, roughly 2 miles into the hike, you'll notice a sudden change in vegetation: The cacti and ocotillo disappear, and you're walking through open grasslands. The trail is narrow but clear and ascends gently, with a few flattish stretches. Occasional bushes and small trees attract birds, making these grasslands far from monotonous, but the trail lacks obvious landmarks such as creek crossings or signposts.

Roughly 4 miles into the hike, at about 5,300 feet elevation, comes the first of several small but noticeable drops in the trail, and the going gets harder. Bordered by small but viciously sharp agave plants, the path becomes indistinct, though little cairns come through as guides. Bushes and small trees such as oaks, junipers, madrones, and pines start becoming a more important part of the landscape.

At this point you could decide upon your own trail end and head back, because you'll have seen all the best views. But if you find it somehow unsatisfying to turn around without having reached some kind of destination, you'll certainly enjoy pushing on along the rough trail. Few people hike up here; I saw no one on my last two hikes. As long as you keep your eyes open for cairns where needed, you'll have no problem in reaching the signpost for the Juniper Basin campsite, just a few feet short of the 6,000-foot-elevation mark. There are no views here, except for the surrounding junipers; the three simple campsites (which require free permits from the visitor center) share a couple of metal bearproof boxes for food storage and have fire rings. The signed toilet is no longer here—perhaps it will be reconstructed someday.

As you enter the campsite, a small seep provides unreliable water in wetter months but dries out for much of the year. A sign indicates that it's 2.1 miles farther to Tanque Verde Peak, the highest point on the ridge at 7,049 feet. Strong hikers could continue to the peak and return for an 18-mile out-and-back trip. The trail to the peak is no more difficult than it has been thus far. The return along the way you came seems easier, not only because you're descending but also because you can see the trail crossing the bare rocky patches, more clearly looking down than looking up.

Nearby Attractions

The **Pima Air and Space Museum** (6000 E. Valencia Rd., Tucson; 520-574-0462; **pimaair.org**) exhibits more than 300 aircraft (and a few rockets) in a mainly outdoor setting. Exhibits range from WWII planes to JFK's *Air Force One* (which can be entered). Open daily, 9 a.m.–5 p.m.; admission is $15.50, with many discounts available. Adjoining the museum, **Davis-Monthan Air Force Base** is home to the 4,200 mothballed military aircraft locally known as "The Boneyard." Guided bus tours are offered for $7, Monday–Friday; call the museum for hours. Drive along Kolb Road between Escalante and Valencia Roads to appreciate this strange sight for free.

See Freeman Homestead Trail (Hike 3, page 45) for details about the visitor center, 1.6 miles away.

Directions

From central Tucson, take 22nd Street east to Old Spanish Trail, which is 0.2 mile east of Harrison Road. Bear right onto Old Spanish Trail, following it southeast for 4 miles to the park entrance and visitor center. Shortly past the visitor center, Cactus Forest Drive forks—take the right fork 1.6 miles to the trailhead.

Coming from the northwest, take 1-10 to Exit 259 and drive east on 22nd Street for 11.3 miles to Old Spanish Trail; then continue as above. Coming from the southeast, take I-10 to Exit 275 and drive north on Houghton Road for 8 miles to Escalante Road. Turn right (east) on Escalante and drive 2 miles to Old Spanish Trail, where you turn left and drive north 0.3 mile to the park entrance.

6

Zimmerman Trailhead to Three Bridges

SCENERY: ★ ★ ★ ★
TRAIL CONDITION: ★ ★ ★
CHILDREN: ★ ★ ★ ★
DIFFICULTY: ★ ★
SOLITUDE: ★ ★ ★ ★

THE GABE ZIMMERMAN MEMORIAL GATE

GPS TRAILHEAD COORDINATES: N32° 00.831' W110° 38.849'

DISTANCE AND CONFIGURATION: 1.8-mile loop

HIKING TIME: 1 hour

HIGHLIGHTS: Trains, bridges, riparian preserve

ELEVATION: 3,435' at trailhead, 3,325' at Cienega Creek

ACCESS: Open 24/7; no fees or permits required for trail use; permit required for hiking off-trail

MAPS: Arizona National Scenic Trail *Passage 8: Rincon Valley* (free PDF at **tinyurl.com /aztpassage8**)

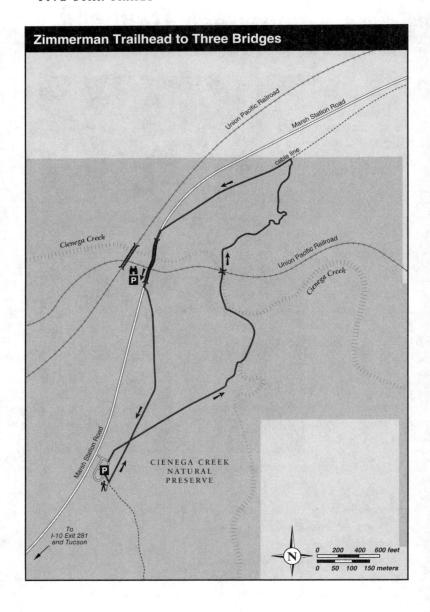

Zimmerman Trailhead to Three Bridges

Union Pacific Railroad

Marsh Station Road

cable line

Cienega Creek

Union Pacific Railroad

Cienega Creek

Marsh Station Road

CIENEGA CREEK
NATURAL
PRESERVE

To
I-10 Exit 281
and Tucson

0   200   400   600 feet

0   50   100   150 meters

N

FACILITIES: Large parking area with 1 picnic table

WHEELCHAIR ACCESS: From trailhead about 0.1 mile to a memorial view bench

COMMENTS: This is part of the Arizona National Scenic Trail. Horses, mountain bikes, and leashed dogs are allowed.

CONTACTS: Arizona Trail Association, 602-252-4794, **aztrail.org;** Pima County Natural Resources, Parks and Recreation, 520-877-6158, **pima.gov/nrpr**

Overview

This short loop begins in the desert and drops quickly into Davidson Canyon, which features the lush and protected riparian habitat of Cienega Creek Natural Preserve. Three bridges jostle for space over Cienega Creek—two carry Union Pacific Railroad trains, and the third is for Marsh Station Road (called Frontage Road or Pantano Road on older maps). It's an unusual synthesis of technology and nature that few people get to appreciate.

Route Details

The trailhead formerly named for Davidson Canyon was officially renamed in 2012 to honor Gabriel "Gabe" Zimmerman (1980–2011), who was an active user of this part of the Arizona Trail. Zimmerman, an aide to U.S. Representative Gabrielle Giffords, was one of six people killed on January 8, 2011, when a gunman opened fire while the congresswoman was conducting a meet-and-greet with Tucson voters. Thirteen people were injured, most seriously Giffords, who resigned from her position and continues to work on her recovery while frequently making appearances in support of issues important to her.

The trailhead features a pedestrian- and wheelchair-accessible gate with a life-size plaque of Gabe Zimmerman. Walk a few steps south-southeast on a paved trail to the intersection with the Arizona National Scenic Trail (AZT), where you turn sharply left (north). Before continuing north, check out the photo plaque just beyond the intersection, which identifies the Rincon Mountains to the north and lists the names of the 19 dead and injured victims of the 2011 shooting. Nearby is a wheelchair-accessible viewpoint of the area.

The AZT goes north along a straight, wide, rocky path following an underground cable line. After 0.1 mile the trail forks, and you follow the small sign to the right (northeast) for the AZT. The trail descends gently through mixed desert vegetation, with various kinds of small cacti scattered through ocotillos and creosote bushes. Crush a couple of creosote leaves to appreciate the pungent odor that these bushes release after a monsoon rain.

Within a few hundred yards, you'll see the green swath of trees of Davidson Canyon below you. The trail becomes narrow and drops easily into the wide bed of Cienega Creek, which is dry for much of the year; however, the 15-foot-high packed-earth banks on either side attest to centuries of flow in the past, and you should be prepared for a creek crossing after heavy rains.

The trail follows the creek bottom as it meanders left (west, then north again) through mature stands of Arizona sycamore, aspens, cottonwoods, and other trees. This is an excellent area for bird-watching. Occasional posts with AZT signs indicate the route along Cienega Creek, and hiking here does not require a permit. The rest of the creek is part of a natural preserve, and you'll need a free permit from Pima County to visit it (see "Contacts").

Soon you'll see bridge trestles bizarrely towering high above the creek. From this angle it's hard to tell why the bridge was built, but if you wait awhile you'll discover that this is a railroad bridge carrying westbound Union Pacific trains. Most of them are long and colorful freight trains coming through numerous times a day; Amtrak rolls past three times a week on its New Orleans–Los Angeles *Sunset Limited* route. True to its name, this train passes through just after the sun goes down, so you probably won't see it.

The trail dips under the bridge and continues about 100 yards past it to an unsigned gap on the right bank of the creek. You might see a pile of rocks or a ribbon here. You've hiked just 0.6 mile from the trailhead.

Climb northeast through the gap in the bank and follow it as it makes a couple of switchbacks to the flatlands above. Two more bridges come into view to the west. The highest and largest is the eastbound Union Pacific railroad bridge; below it is the light-colored bridge carrying Marsh Station Road vehicular traffic over the creek. Look south to glimpse traffic on the I-10 freeway, almost 2 miles away, and farther south to views of the Santa Rita Mountains and the Whetstone Mountains to the southeast.

The trail reaches the cable line and turns sharply left (west), reaching Marsh Station Road after 0.2 mile. At the road you can return the way you came, 2.7 miles out-and-back, or continue left to the parking lot for a 1.8-mile loop. The AZT crosses the road and continues under the eastbound railroad bridge high on the right side of Cienega Creek. Our trail back to the parking lot necessitates crossing the Marsh Station Road bridge, which does not have a pedestrian walkway. Traffic is sparse, and with care you should be able to cross without a problem.

The far end of the bridge crosses over the westbound railway tracks. Immediately past the road bridge, on the right side, is a brightly colored sign for the Cienega Creek Natural Preserve and a small parking area for AZT users. This is also an excellent observation point for train aficionados. Opposite the sign, on the left side of the road, a short dirt road leads down to the railway tracks and a trail follows the cable line to the south-southeast. Hike along this trail a few minutes to return to the Gabe Zimmerman Trailhead.

Directions

Drive east on I-10 to Exit 281/AZ 83, roughly 20 miles east of Tucson. Immediately after leaving the freeway, turn left over the freeway and follow a sign for Frontage Road to Marsh Station Road. Turn right, then right again, onto Marsh Station Road, and drive 3 miles to the Gabe Zimmerman Trailhead parking area, on your right.

OCOTILLOS FLOWER IN MAY ON THE TANQUE VERDE RIDGE TRAIL.

(See Hike 5, page 59.)

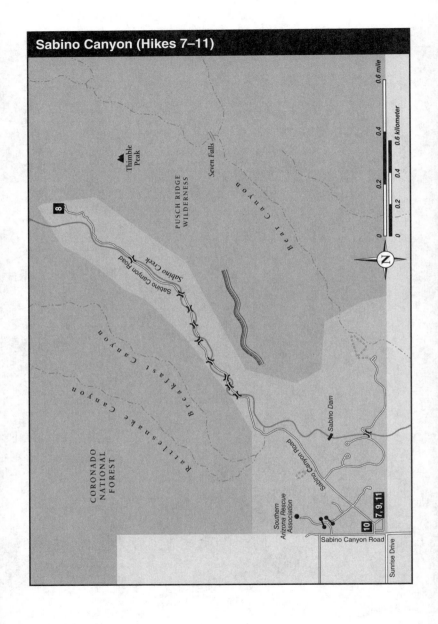

Sabino Canyon (Hikes 7–11)

Thimble Peak

PUSCH RIDGE WILDERNESS

Seven Falls

Bear Canyon

8

Sabino Canyon Road

Sabino Creek

Breakfast Canyon

Rattlesnake Canyon

CORONADO NATIONAL FOREST

Sabino Dam

Sabino Canyon Road

Southern Arizona Rescue Association

7, 9, 11

10

Sabino Canyon Road

Sunrise Drive

N

| 0 | 0.2 | 0.4 | 0.6 kilometer |

| 0 | 0.2 | 0.4 | 0.6 mile |

Sabino Canyon

YELLOW BRITTLEBUSH FLOWERS SURROUND HEDGEHOG CACTUS BLOOMS.

Blackett's Ridge Trail

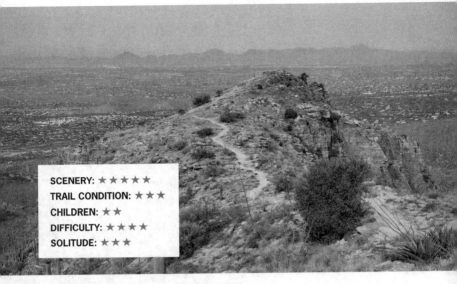

SCENERY: ★ ★ ★ ★ ★
TRAIL CONDITION: ★ ★ ★
CHILDREN: ★ ★
DIFFICULTY: ★ ★ ★ ★
SOLITUDE: ★ ★ ★

VIEW OF TUCSON FROM BLACKETT'S RIDGE

GPS TRAILHEAD COORDINATES: N32° 18.560' W110° 49.317'

DISTANCE AND CONFIGURATION: 6.2-mile out-and-back

HIKING TIME: 3 hours

HIGHLIGHTS: Splendid views of Sabino Canyon from vertical cliffs; Bear Canyon and city views; bird-watching; a good workout

ELEVATION: 2,725' at parking lot, 4,409' at trail's end

ACCESS: Open 24/7; parking $5/$10/$20 for day/week/year; all National Park Service annual passes accepted

MAPS: Green Trails *Map 2886S–Santa Catalina Mountains,* USFS *Pusch Ridge Wilderness,* USGS *Sabino Canyon;* free map at visitor center

FACILITIES: Visitor center, flush toilets, vending machines

WHEELCHAIR ACCESS: Visitor center, toilets, Sabino Canyon Road (page 91), and the first 0.8 mile of the trail (requires some pushes)

COMMENTS: No pets; no bicycles; horses permitted but rarely encountered. Large parking lot fills by mid-morning on spring weekends—if you park on the road outside, you risk a ticket. (However, if you drive 0.2 mile north on Sabino Canyon Road, past the No Parking signs, you can park and walk back.) The last trail section is signed and mapped as 1.7 miles, but I measured it at about 1.3 miles on my GPS. (It certainly *felt* like 1.7!)

CONTACTS: Sabino Canyon Visitor Center, 520-749-8700, **www.fs.usda.gov/coronado**

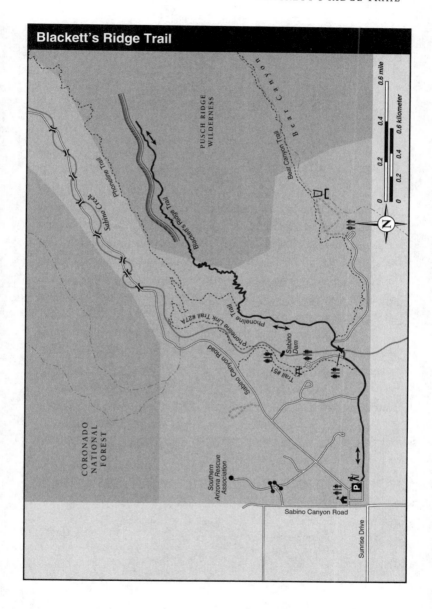

Blackett's Ridge Trail

Overview

Some Tucsonans take a masochistic pleasure in running up this steep trail and pride themselves on getting to the summit in well under an hour from the parking lot. Others claim to climb it most days of the week to stay in shape. I prefer to take my time to enjoy the best views in Sabino Canyon and keep an eye out for the flora and fauna.

Route Details

From the southeast end of the parking lot, the trail follows the same route as the Phoneline Trail (page 85) for the first 1.4 miles until it reaches a junction signed "Blackett's Ridge Trail #48 1.7 Miles to End of Trail." From 1937 and into the 1940s, a teacher at the Southern Arizona School for Boys named Don Everett used to explore this area on foot and horseback, accompanied by some of his students. He would label unnamed landmarks after some of his boys—in this case after a student named Blackett.

At the junction, turn east (right), and within a few yards you'll see a table-sized flat boulder shaded by a mesquite tree on the right side of the trail. You're just 300 feet in elevation above the parking lot, so this rock is a good place to sit and consider whether you have enough water and stamina to climb the steep 1,400 feet from here to the top.

The trail starts climbing moderately for a few hundred yards and then begins a series of steep switchbacks up the western nose of the ridge. Sometimes I've been accompanied by a raven that likes to hang out around these steep rocks. During the summer, lizards abound and occasional snakes and Gila monsters show up on the sharp, rocky, narrow trail.

After 15–20 minutes of climbing, watch for a flat area on the left side, which gives you a chance to step off the trail and admire the burgeoning view of Tucson to the west and Sabino Canyon to the north and east (your left). Above you are two or three convenient flattish areas to break your hike, all with fine views, so don't feel that you need to stop in the middle of the narrow trail for a drink of water.

Because this trail is short and steep, you'll find that the plant life varies both with elevation and time of year. What you may see at 3,000 feet elevation arrives later at 4,000 feet.

Look for small blue, yellow, white, and orange desert flowers in March; palo verde trees densely blossoming yellow in April; and ocotillos showing off red flowers into May, when saguaros join in with their white blooms. Into the hot months of June and July, many agaves along the trail thrust their 20-foot-high spikes into the air, topped with dozens of tight, bowl-like clusters of yellow and orange flowers. Barrel cacti are among the latest of the cacti to bloom, with a ring of golden flowers forming a striking crown.

After the initial series of switchbacks, the obvious trail includes some shorter, flatter sections, and your first views of Bear Canyon appear to the right (south). About halfway up, the trail climbs through some rocky slabs where the route isn't always obvious, but if you simply keep climbing, you'll find the trail within a minute or two. If you don't, look back and around and you should see the route. You have to keep climbing.

Next comes a clear trail heading to a peak—it's false. There are at least two, some folks say three, false summits; I think it depends on how out of breath you feel after this climb. When you come to a narrow ridge with exciting views of Sabino Canyon and Bear Canyon on either side, you'll know you're near the end of the trail. By now, you'll have noticed distinctive Thimble Peak (5,323 feet) on the horizon in front of you, 1.5 miles away to the northeast.

Suddenly, a small marker tells you that you've arrived at the end of the trail. Beyond this sign, you can scramble down a rough path for a couple of hundred feet before it peters out in a frighteningly steep saddle; this area is called Saddleback on many maps.

To your left, the sheer cliffs drop for hundreds of feet, so watch your step. Most of Sabino Canyon Road is visible, with occasional shuttle vehicles crossing the bridges more than 1,000 feet below. From mid-February to mid-October, swallows are commonly seen swooping along the cliff top as they busily capture insects, and hawks and vultures often patrol the area. Enjoy a bird-watching break and then return the way you came.

Nearby Attractions

See Hike 10, Sabino Canyon Road (page 91).

Directions

See Hike 10.

8 Hutch's Pool

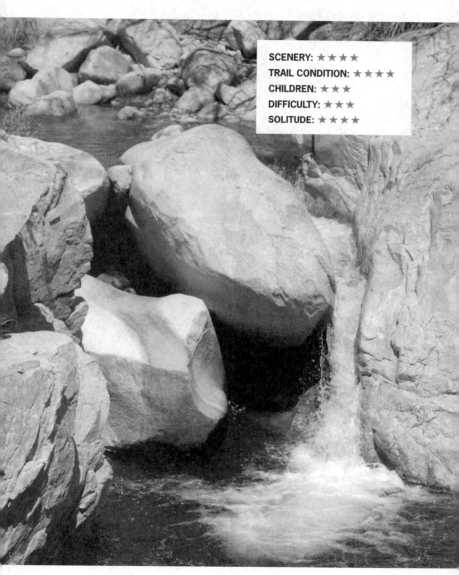

SCENERY: ★ ★ ★ ★
TRAIL CONDITION: ★ ★ ★ ★
CHILDREN: ★ ★ ★
DIFFICULTY: ★ ★ ★
SOLITUDE: ★ ★ ★ ★

HUTCH'S POOL

Sabino Canyon: Hutch's Pool

West Fork Trail

Hutch's
Pool

Sabino Creek

West Fork Trail

CORONADO
NATIONAL
FOREST

PUSCH RIDGE
WILDERNESS

Sabino Creek

Sabino Canyon Trail

Stop
#9

Sabino Canyon Road

Phoneline Trail

N

| 0 | 0.2 | 0.4 | 0.6 mile |

| 0 | 0.2 | 0.4 | 0.6 kilometer |

GPS TRAILHEAD COORDINATES: N32° 20.626' W110° 46.831'

DISTANCE AND CONFIGURATION: 8.2-mile out-and-back using the trailhead shuttle, 15.8-mile out-and-back from the parking lot

HIKING TIME: 4.5 hours

HIGHLIGHTS: Year-round water deep enough to swim in; attractive high-desert scenery

ELEVATION: 3,334' at trailhead, 3,850' at Hutch's Pool

ACCESS: Open 24/7; parking $5/$10/$20 for day/week/year; all National Park Service annual passes accepted

MAPS: Green Trails Map 2886S–Santa Catalina Mountains, USFS Pusch Ridge Wilderness, USGS Sabino Canyon

FACILITIES: Visitor center, flush toilets, vending machines at parking lot; motorized shuttle to trailhead

WHEELCHAIR ACCESS: None on the trail

COMMENTS: No pets. Maps and U.S. Forest Service signs show the distance as 8.2 miles; my GPS showed 7.8 miles. Sabino Canyon Tours runs a motorized shuttle to the trailhead every hour (every 30 minutes on weekends, holidays, and busy days in spring), 9 a.m.–4:30 p.m.; $8, $4 for children ages 3–12, free for kids age 2 and younger. You can reach the trailhead via Sabino Canyon Road (see page 91) and add 7.6 miles out-and-back, or you can join the trail via the Phoneline Trail (see page 85) for longer, all-day hikes.

CONTACTS: Sabino Canyon Visitor Center, 520-749-8700, **www.fs.usda.gov/coronado;** Sabino Canyon Tours, 520-749-2861, **sabinocanyon.com**

Overview

Hutch's Pool comes a distinct second to Seven Falls as a destination for water-seeking hikers in the Sabino Canyon area, but it ranks first as a year-round water attraction—it doesn't dry up completely. The first section from the trailhead, the only steep one, is rewarded with great views back down Sabino Canyon. Continuing on, the trail encounters a variety of landscapes, including a steep canyon and high desert grasslands.

Route Details

Beginning from the last shuttle stop, Sabino Canyon Trail #23 climbs via wide stairs to . . . hey, not so fast. On a recent hike I almost stepped on a rattlesnake curled up on the stairs, less than 100 yards away

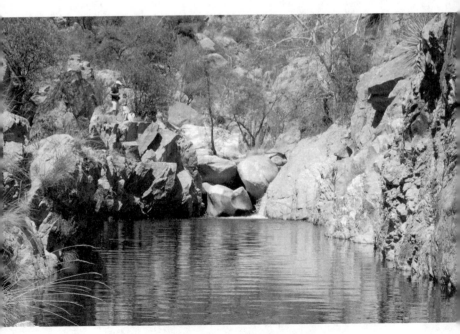

BEAUTIFUL HUTCH'S POOL IS A POPULAR SWIMMING HOLE.

from the end of the road. I waited awhile and then walked around what I guessed to be the back of the snake—hard to tell when they're coiled up. You need to keep your eyes open, even if you just got off the shuttle. Of course, I've hiked on these stairs many times without seeing a rattler, so you shouldn't think this particular trail is any more likely to provide you with a snake sighting. That could happen on almost any hike in this book, so be aware.

Climb almost 0.5 mile on well-graded stairs and switchbacks to the intersection with Phoneline Trail #27. This short section is the most heavily used, with shuttle riders experiencing a taste of desert hiking and Phoneline Trail users making a final descent to the road. The views back down Sabino Canyon, with the Phoneline Trail clinging high to the left side, are increasingly impressive as you climb. At the junction, make a hard left to continue northwest along the Sabino Canyon Trail.

The trail continues to climb, but the switchbacks become less frequent. After 0.4 mile the route flattens and follows high up the right-hand side of the canyon, with good views of the canyon below and glimpses of Sabino Creek. After a few hundred flat yards, the trail crosses over the top of a large rock outcrop, then diverges away from the canyon to the east, passing through a landscape of grasses, bushes, spring flowers, and occasional yuccas and agaves, but relatively few cacti.

Soon the trail swings back to the north, still mainly flat; about 1 mile from the rock outcrop, it begins to drop toward an intersection of streams coming from several small canyons and flowing into Sabino Creek. A sign indicates West Fork Trail #24, where you turn left (north-northwest) and cross Box Canyon Stream, seeking cairns to guide you. Boulders in the stream may help keep your feet dry if the water is flowing high.

Beyond the stream, the trail heads generally west and, after a few hundred yards, switchbacks suddenly and turns north briefly before continuing west-northwest through golden fields of poppies in March and April, or grasslands and bushes the rest of the year. A few hundred yards farther, you'll pass a football field–sized flat area to your left that has stone fire rings where people have camped. Sabino Creek is nearby. Beyond, the trail enters thick riparian woodlands and follows the right bank of the creek. Canyons, streams, grasslands, and now woodlands—this hike certainly offers variety.

Roughly 1.25 miles along the West Fork Trail, cross to the left bank of Sabino Creek, using stepping-stones or possibly wading after monsoon storms. Cairns show the route. Continue on the left bank for 0.3 mile and look for a 1.5-foot-tall pile of rocks on the right of the trail: This marks the turnoff to Hutch's Pool, barely 100 yards away but not visible from the West Fork Trail. If you miss the turnoff and start climbing steeply, you'll be on the 5-mile-long trail to Romero Pass, so go back and look again.

The year-round pool is hidden in a secluded slot canyon, with a tiny beach for wading at the south end and small cliffs and a pretty little waterfall at the north end, where the water is reportedly up to 15 feet deep—check first before plunging in. In winter and spring the water is bracingly cold, but it warms to just-right in summer, when the hike is extremely hot (carry plenty of water). At any time, this attractive high desert pool makes an excellent destination for lunch, after which you return the way you came.

Nearby Attractions

See Hike 10, Sabino Canyon Road (page 91).

Directions

Follow the directions for Hike 10. After you park, either take the shuttle or walk 3.7 miles up Sabino Canyon Road to the trailhead.

Phoneline Trail

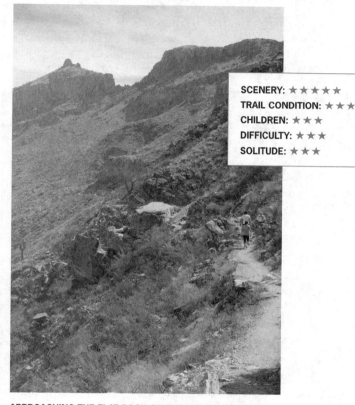

SCENERY: ★ ★ ★ ★ ★
TRAIL CONDITION: ★ ★ ★ ★
CHILDREN: ★ ★ ★
DIFFICULTY: ★ ★ ★
SOLITUDE: ★ ★ ★

APPROACHING THE FLAT ROCK ON THE PHONELINE TRAIL

GPS TRAILHEAD COORDINATES: N32° 18.560' W110° 49.317'

DISTANCE AND CONFIGURATION: 4-mile short loop, 11-mile out-and-back, or 5.5-mile point-to-point and return on Sabino Canyon Road hike or shuttle

HIKING TIME: 1.75 hours for short loop, 5 hours for out-and-back, 4 hours to hike out and return along Sabino Canyon Road

HIGHLIGHTS: Saguaros galore, spring flowers, and soaring canyon views, plus creek and dam views on the short loop

ELEVATION: 2,725' at parking lot, 3,190' at high point on short loop, 3,660' at high point on out-and-back

ACCESS: Open 24/7; parking $5/$10/$20 for day/week/year; all National Park Service annual passes accepted

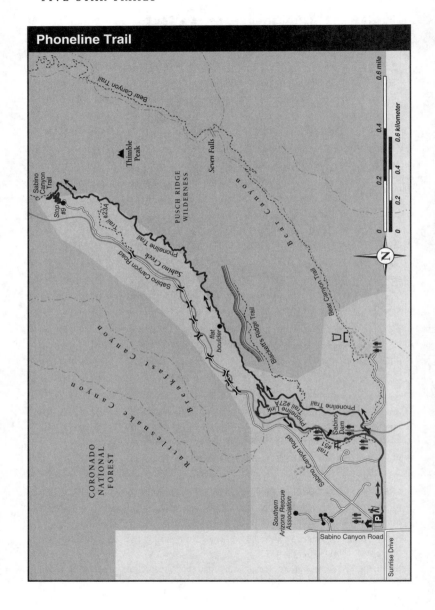

Phoneline Trail

MAPS: Green Trails *Map 2886S–Santa Catalina Mountains*, USFS *Pusch Ridge Wilderness*, USGS *Sabino Canyon*; free map at visitor center

FACILITIES: Visitor center, flush toilets, vending machines

WHEELCHAIR ACCESS: Visitor center, toilets, Sabino Canyon Road (page 91), and the first 0.8 mile of the trail (requires some pushes)

COMMENTS: No pets, no bicycles, horses permitted but rarely encountered. Large parking lot fills by mid-morning on spring weekends—if you park on the road outside, you risk a ticket. (However, if you drive 0.2 mile north on Sabino Canyon Road, past the No Parking signs, you can park and walk back.)

CONTACTS: Sabino Canyon Visitor Center, 520-749-8700, **www.fs.usda.gov/coronado**

Overview

When I have out-of-town guests who want a fun hike where they can see plenty of saguaros and great desert and canyon scenery without taking up too much time and energy, I inevitably take them on the shortened loop of the Phoneline Link Trail. Everyone loves it. With a bit more time on one's hands, the complete Phoneline Trail—hanging dramatically between cliff top and canyon bottom—makes a hiker feel like an eagle soaring in and out of gullies. Some hikers take the Sabino Canyon shuttle (see page 93) to the end of Sabino Canyon Road and hike the Phoneline Trail in reverse.

Route Details

From the southeast end of the parking lot, the trail begins with a sign for Bear Canyon Trailhead, adjacent to a map and a drinking fountain. Walk east on a flat track wide enough to hike six abreast. After about 100 yards, the optional 0.25-mile Bajada Loop Nature Trail is to the left. It's wheelchair-accessible but unpaved, so helpful pushes may be needed to enjoy this educational experience.

The wide track terminates at Bear Canyon Road, almost 0.5 mile from the parking lot. Follow the road to your right for 0.25 mile until you reach a restroom (flush toilets, drinking water), which you should consider using because the Phoneline Trail is narrow and exposed with no convenient bushes. Stop 2 on the Bear Canyon shuttle route is outside the restroom. Here, turn right (east), following the sign for Sabino Dam East and Bear Canyon. The road crosses a bridge over Sabino Creek—a bridge that can be knee-deep in overflowing water during spring runoffs or autumn monsoons. In that case, take your boots off and wade carefully across. Usually, the creek trickles pleasantly under the bridge, but it dries up completely in summer.

Immediately past the bridge, the road comes to a T-junction; cross the junction to find a sign for Phoneline Trail #27. Climb the narrow, rocky trail, and almost immediately find another signed T-junction, where you turn left and start climbing steadily east and swinging quickly to the north. You are following the route of the historic phone line that used to be the main link between Tucson and the Palisade Ranger Station on Mount Lemmon before the road now known as the Catalina Highway was built.

The climb is gentle—about 500 feet of elevation gain in almost a mile—but provides increasingly open views of the saguaro forest and, in spring, wildflowers. Almost 0.6 mile along the trail, a signed junction to the right (east) indicates the Blackett's Ridge Trail (page 74). The Phoneline Trail continues northeast and then swings dramatically around to the northwest, hugging the canyon contours.

Views of Sabino Canyon Road below and downtown Tucson, 11 miles away to the southwest, become increasingly grand until you reach a trail fork 0.4 mile beyond the Blackett's Ridge junction. Here, you have the choice of continuing along the main Phoneline Trail to your right or taking the Phoneline Link Trail #27A to your left—the latter is the shortened loop, described later in this section.

The Phoneline Trail is clear but narrow, with nowhere to step off, climbing gently northeast with increasingly splendid views of the canyon. To the left of the trail, the canyon wall tumbles steeply to the road hundreds of feet below, and to the right it climbs to the canyon top, so looking for a place to take a break is exceedingly difficult. Look for a semi trailer–sized flat boulder on the left side after about 0.7 mile—it makes a great place to stop for a snack while thinking about how and when this massive piece of rock detached itself from the cliffs above. Onward, the airy route swoops and slants like a hawk, following the contours of the canyon until it reaches the intersection with the Historic Sabino Trail #23A, 2 miles beyond the flat boulder. Here, you could descend steeply on a rough and rocky 0.7-mile trail to Sabino Canyon Road (page 91), reaching the road just above Bridge 9 and below Shuttle Stop 8.

Continuing on the main Phoneline Trail for another 0.5 mile brings you to the junction with Sabino Canyon Trail #23. At this point, you could turn around and return the way you came, saving yourself the final steep section, or turn left and zigzag steeply down for 0.5 mile to the end of Sabino Canyon Road at Shuttle Stop 9. Here, continue down Sabino Canyon Road to the visitor center, or retrace your hike on the Phoneline Trail.

The **Phoneline Link Trail #27A** makes a convenient descent for the shortened loop, switchbacking toward the road below. After 0.6 mile, you'll reach a trail junction marked "Creek Trail #52," where you turn left. (If you turn right, you'll cross Sabino Creek, which can be dry or knee-deep depending on the season, to reach Sabino Canyon Road at Shuttle Stop 1, just 0.1 mile away.)

Creek Trail doesn't have many water views, meandering instead through desert woodland of mesquite and palo verde trees, often accompanied by birdsong. After 0.2 mile, Creek Trail crosses a sandy wash that's almost always dry—look for the brown trail marker on the other side. The trail follows the right side of the wash for 0.1 mile and then crosses it again; look for stones marking the way. Another 0.1 mile brings you to an unsigned fork. Going left takes you along the left bank of Sabino Creek, and you arrive at the east side of small Sabino Dam after 0.2 mile. Going right crosses the creek (you might have to wade) and gets you to the west side of the dam. This side also gives access to Bluff Trail #51, leading to Sabino Canyon Road (0.2 mile) and other trails paralleling the main trail.

Above the dam is so-called Sabino Lake, which is dry in summer and a shallow pond in other months. Below the dam, water holes and sliding rocks are popular with kids in spring and fall, but dry in summer. Whichever side of the dam you end up on, continue about 0.3 mile to the road bridge that you crossed near the beginning of the hike, and return along the road and wide, flat track to the parking area.

Nearby Attractions

See next hike.

Directions

See next hike.

10

Sabino Canyon Road

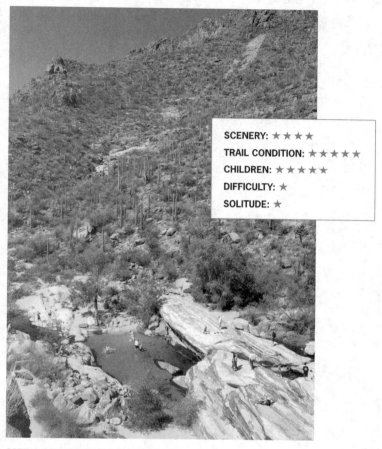

SCENERY: ★ ★ ★ ★
TRAIL CONDITION: ★ ★ ★ ★ ★
CHILDREN: ★ ★ ★ ★ ★
DIFFICULTY: ★
SOLITUDE: ★

SABINO CANYON POOLS BY SHUTTLE STOP 8

GPS TRAILHEAD COORDINATES: N32° 18.600' W110° 49.359'
DISTANCE AND CONFIGURATION: 7.6-mile out-and-back
HIKING TIME: 2.5 hours
HIGHLIGHTS: Seasonal swimming holes; canyon views; family-friendly
ELEVATION: 2,725' at visitor center, 3,350' at trail's end
ACCESS: Open 24/7; parking $5/$10/$20 for day/week/year; all National Park Service annual passes accepted

Sabino Canyon Road

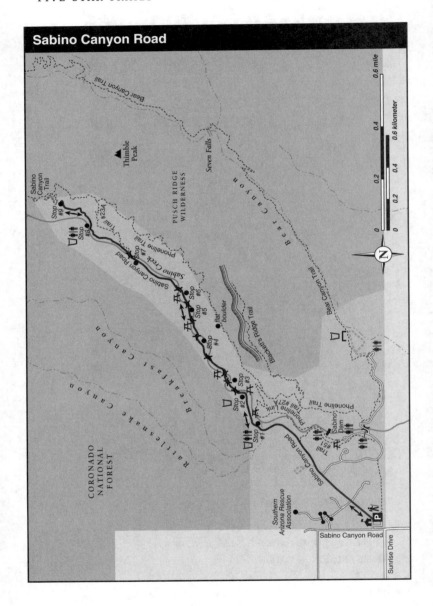

MAPS: Green Trails *Map 2886S–Santa Catalina Mountains*, USFS *Pusch Ridge Wilderness*, USGS *Sabino Canyon*; free map at visitor center. Note, though, that this is one of the few hikes you can do without a map—you can't get lost on the road.

FACILITIES: Visitor center, flush toilets, vending machines, motorized shuttle

WHEELCHAIR ACCESS: The entire road is wheelchair-accessible.

COMMENTS: Best wheelchair hike. Bicycles permitted daily, 5 p.m.–9 a.m., except Wednesday and Saturday. No pets. Sabino Canyon Tours runs a motorized shuttle every hour (every 30 minutes on weekends and holidays), 9 a.m.–4.30 p.m.; $8, $4 for children ages 3–12, free for kids age 2 and younger. Large parking lot fills by mid-morning on spring weekends—if you park on the road outside, you risk a ticket. (However, if you drive 0.2 mile north on Sabino Canyon Road, past the No Parking signs, you can park and walk back.)

CONTACTS: Sabino Canyon Visitor Center, 520-749-8700, **www.fs.usda.gov/coronado**; Sabino Canyon Tours, 520-749-2861, **sabinocanyon.com**

Overview

This paved road is closed to vehicles (except for limited bicycle and shuttle traffic) and provides walkers, joggers, parents with strollers, and folks in wheelchairs with a gorgeous hiking experience—it's the best place in Tucson to get into the wilderness with a wheelchair. The tour shuttle has a flat fee that allows all-day on-and-off privileges at any of its nine stops, and can be used to access the Hutch's Pool Trail (page 79) or to hike the Phoneline Trail (page 85) in reverse.

Route Details

With its nine single-lane bridges crossing Sabino Creek, Sabino Canyon Road was a civil construction project in the 1930s, and some of the blocky bridge architecture echoes that era. Tucson families used to drive up here to take advantage of the cool water holes until the road was closed in the 1970s. Today the road remains in great condition (for the open-air shuttles) and accesses plenty of swimming holes and picnic sites near the bridges and shuttle stops. The best time to go for a dip is spring and fall—the creek dries up in summer (mid-May–August) and is icy-cold in winter.

Begin hiking on the road, heading straight (northeast) from the shuttle-ticket booth. Just past the shade ramada behind the ticket booth on the right side of the road, you'll see a foot trail that parallels the road for about 0.5 mile. Most people walk the road, but you can take the parallel trail, just a stone's throw away. Even though you're just a few steps from the parking lot and visitor center, keep your eyes open for wildlife ranging from roadrunners to deer. A mountain lion was seen and photographed near the lower part of the road in 2013. Look up to the right of the road for views of Blackett's Ridge (page 74).

After 0.5 mile, the road to Bear Canyon (page 97) goes to the right—keep going straight (northeast), climbing gently and then dropping slightly. To your right, 0.8 mile along the road, Trail #51 heads to Sabino Dam (see previous hike). Enjoy views of the cottonwood trees in Sabino Creek, golden in fall and into the mild winter. Shuttle Stop 1 is between two restrooms on the right, 1.2 miles along the road; there are picnic tables by the second restroom, which has a drinking fountain and wheelchair-accessible flush toilets and picnic tables. Trail #27A starts from here, climbing to the Phoneline Trail.

By now you're in Sabino Canyon proper, with cliffs rising on both sides. Occasional short trails lead down from the right of the road to picnic areas by Sabino Creek, just a few yards away. Shuttle Stop 2 is 1.5 miles along the road; this has the last potable water until Stop 8. Soon after Stop 2, the road crosses the first of nine bridges along

Sabino Creek. (Note that the shuttle stops have numbered signs, but you'll have to count the nine bridges for yourself.) Pools and a diminutive waterfall invite kids to play, but don't feel that you need to stop here—plenty of other riparian areas are farther along the road.

After Stop 2 is the second bridge, with a couple of picnic tables nearby. At the end of the bridge, on the right, is a fine example of an Arizona sycamore tree, with its pale, flaky-looking bark. Soon you'll see Thimble Peak—it really does look like a thimble!—rising on the horizon, dead ahead as you walk. To your right, Acropolis Wall is the cliff rising more than 400 feet straight up to Blackett's Ridge. You'll continue crossing bridge after bridge, with shuttle stop after shuttle stop; most have no or very basic facilities, but you can explore spots to dip your toes at every creek crossing.

Soon after Stop 7 (2.9 miles), you'll cross the ninth and last bridge on the road. A few yards farther, on the right, a sign indicates Trail #23A, which climbs, rockily and steeply, to connect with the Phoneline Trail 0.7 mile away.

Stop 8, at mile 3.2, offers a water fountain and vault toilets. Stairs at the end of a parking area lead down to Sabino Creek, now to your left, and a trail leads upriver to numerous popular swimming holes, tanning rocks, and cascades. From Stop 8, it's another 0.5 mile to the end of the road at Stop 9, which is the trailhead of the hike to Hutch's Pool (see page 79) or the Phoneline Trail (see page 85) in reverse. The only facilities here are benches; there was a restroom here until July 31, 2006, when a memorably massive monsoon storm caused rockslides in the upper canyon that washed away the entire facility and parts of the road.

Nearby Attractions

The **Sabino Canyon Visitor Center,** open daily, 8.30 a.m.–4.30 p.m., has information and useful free brochures. It also offers a small but interesting exhibit about the history, geology, and wildlife of the canyon, a short movie in the theater, and a gift shop with a fine selection of maps, books, and Sabino Canyon paraphernalia. The visitor center is also the Coronado National Forest Ranger Station; the rangers can answer questions about Mount Lemmon and the Catalina Foothills, all of which lie within the forest.

Directions

From central Tucson, take Broadway or Speedway Boulevard east to Wilmot Road. Turn left on Wilmot, which veers right at Pima Street and becomes Tanque Verde Road. Travel east on Tanque Verde for 1 mile and turn left on Sabino Canyon Road. Follow Sabino Canyon Road about 5 miles to Sabino Canyon, on your right.

From I-10, coming from the southeast, take Exit 270/Kolb Road and follow it north for 10.5 miles to Tanque Verde Road. Turn right on Tanque Verde and, after 0.5 mile, turn left on Sabino Canyon Road; follow it about 5 miles to Sabino Canyon, on your right.

From I-10, coming from the northwest, take Exit 248/Ina Road and head east. After 6.8 miles, Ina becomes Skyline Drive and, almost 2 miles farther, becomes Sunrise Drive. Follow Sunrise about 7 miles until it dead-ends at Sabino Canyon Road. Turn left; Sabino Canyon is the first entrance on your right.

11 Seven Falls on
Bear Canyon Trail

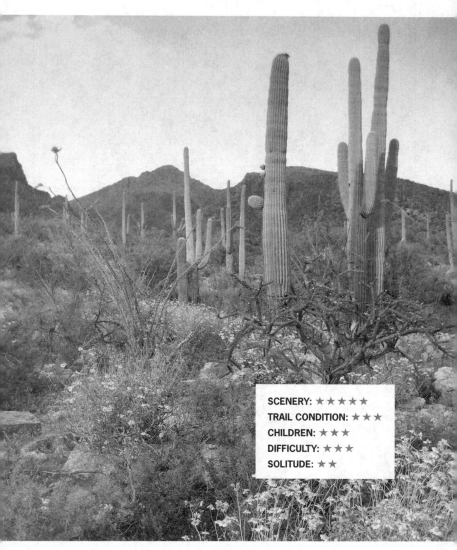

SCENERY: ★ ★ ★ ★ ★
TRAIL CONDITION: ★ ★ ★
CHILDREN: ★ ★ ★
DIFFICULTY: ★ ★ ★
SOLITUDE: ★ ★

RED OCOTILLO BLOOMS ABOVE YELLOW BRITTLEBUSH.

Seven Falls on Bear Canyon Trail

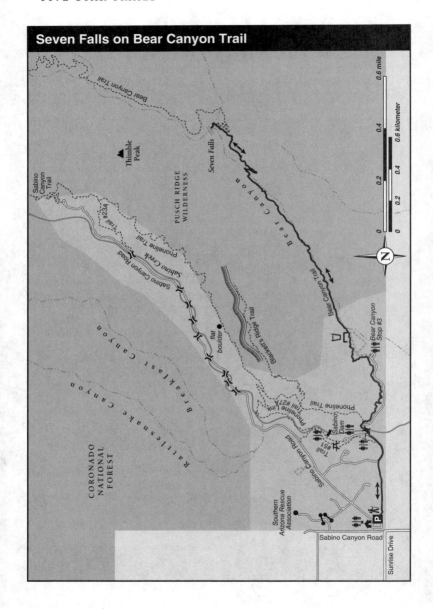

GPS TRAILHEAD COORDINATES: N32° 18.560' W110° 49.317'

DISTANCE AND CONFIGURATION: 7.8-mile out-and-back, 5-mile out-and-back using the Bear Canyon shuttle

HIKING TIME: 3–5 hours for the whole hike (depending on water levels)

HIGHLIGHTS: Lovely views at Seven Falls with cooling pools below

ELEVATION: 2,725' at parking lot, 3,440' at high point, 3,300' at base of falls

ACCESS: Open 24/7; parking $5/$10/$20 for day/week/year; all National Park Service annual passes accepted

MAPS: Green Trails Map 2886S–*Santa Catalina Mountains*, USFS *Pusch Ridge Wilderness*, USGS *Sabino Canyon*; free map at visitor center

FACILITIES: Visitor center, flush toilets, vending machines. Sabino Canyon Tours runs a motorized shuttle to Bear Canyon hourly, 9 a.m.–4 p.m.; $3, $1 for children ages 3–12, free for kids age 2 and younger.

WHEELCHAIR ACCESS: Visitor center, toilets, Sabino Canyon Road (page 91), and the first 1.4 miles of the trail (requires some pushes on the unpaved parts)

COMMENTS: No pets; bicycles permitted on paved Bear Canyon Road daily, 5 p.m.– 9 a.m., except Wednesday and Saturday; horses permitted but rarely encountered. The Bear Canyon shuttle takes a different route for most of the way to the Seven Falls trailhead.

CONTACTS: Sabino Canyon Visitor Center, 520-749-8700, **www.fs.usda.gov/coronado**; Sabino Canyon Tours, 520-749-2861, **sabinocanyon.com**

Overview

This trail is a rite of passage for young Tucsonans and University of Arizona students for whom the Seven Falls take on an almost-mythical status. During weekends in spring and fall, flat rocks and shallow pools at the base of the falls are surrounded by scores of semi-clad sunbathers, some of whom scramble up unsanctioned routes on either side of the lower falls. The ribbon-like cascades aren't very big, even after rains, but there are seven of them if you count the one below the pools, and they certainly are attractive when in full spate. From mid-May to July, the falls dry out completely.

The trail crosses Bear Creek seven times en route to the falls. When it's dry the crossings are easy, but in high water you may have to wade knee-deep or look for boulders to jump across on, which means that finding the best trail can be time-consuming. Bring a walking stick or trekking pole for greater safety when crossing the water. Ask at the visitor center for current conditions, and beware of flash floods. On August 4, 2007, a monsoonal flood swept through Bear Canyon, forcing dozens of hikers to clamber up the canyon sides to avoid being swept away; lamentably, two young adults drowned, even though they were fit and able to swim.

Route Details

From the southeast end of the parking lot, the trail follows the same route as the Phoneline Trail (page 85) until after the bridge crossing over Sabino Creek, some 0.75 mile from the parking area. Beyond the bridge, the road hits a T-junction and the right turn is signed "Seven Falls." This paved road, which heads briefly south and then east, is the route that the Bear Canyon shuttle takes, and many hikers walk out along it. A more natural alternative is to take the trail, which parallels the road on the north side. This trail shares the Phoneline Trail for about 150 feet, and then a small sign indicates Bear Canyon Trail #29—here, go right (south) for about 200 feet before swinging around to the east.

From the almost-flat trail, you catch glimpses of the road to the right and see Blackett's Ridge rearing up a mile to your left, with several ridges of the Santa Catalina Mountains behind. Flowers abound in spring, and saguaros surround you year-round. You'll meet the paved road after about 0.5 mile. This is where the Bear Canyon Shuttle ends at Stop 3, with a restroom, water, and a shadeless picnic table and barbecue grill. If you're riding the shuttle, make sure you know when the last one leaves for the return journey.

The road continues east but is now unpaved, and the trail continues paralleling it to the north. After 0.4 mile, the unpaved road ends at a ramada with a bench and a water faucet—fill up your water bottles here. From this point, you'll be heading east-northeast on a narrow, rocky, but clear trail following the left side of Bear Creek, which you'll be crossing seven times as you climb gently up the canyon. The first crossing is 0.25 mile from the end of the unpaved road—look for a short flight of rocky steps on the far side of the creek. The crossing is obvious in dry months but can be a challenge during spring runoffs or fall monsoons. If you have any problems wading across in the wet months, you might consider that this is the first of seven crossings!

Most hikers, most of the time, forge on. The first six crossings are clustered together in a 0.6-mile stretch, so if you get your feet wet, you might want to just keep sloshing on rather than drying off every time. The trail is partially shaded by a riparian woodland of willow, ash, and mesquite trees with birds flitting among them, but a glance upward at the walls of Bear Canyon reminds you that you're in the desert.

Half a mile beyond the sixth river crossing, a small sign indicates that the trail drops to the left (north) bank of the creek for a short while. If water levels are high, you might have to scramble over a rough and steep little outcrop. About 300 feet farther you'll come to the seventh crossing, which is the least obvious—hikers often end up missing the right place to cross. Look for a wooden post on the other side of the creek and aim for that.

This crossing is about 3,050 feet elevation, and beyond it the trail starts climbing and switchbacking above the right side of Bear Creek. Eventually it flattens and follows the high right side of the canyon, until you reach a trail fork at about 3,440 feet elevation and 0.5 mile beyond the seventh crossing. Here, take the unsigned left fork, which drops to the base of Seven Falls.

(If you take the right fork, signed "Bear Canyon Trail #29," you'll be in for more than 8 more miles of hiking up to 4,720 feet elevation, then down via East Fork Trail #24A and Sabino Canyon Trail #23 to the top end of Sabino Canyon Road. This enables you to climb Bear Canyon and return via Sabino Canyon Road—an approximately 17-mile hike that is doable in one long day if you're a fit, experienced hiker with a map.)

The short, steep trail to the base of the falls has excellent views of all seven falls—you can't see them properly from the fork. You'll skirt around the right side of the pools at the bottom, and you can make an eighth creek crossing as you explore. Beware of very slippery, algae-covered rocks when the falls are running, and be prepared for dry pools in early summer.

Nearby Attractions

See previous hike.

Directions

See previous hike.

SAGUARO AND SPIRE ON SABINO CANYON TRAIL *(see Hike 8, page 79)*

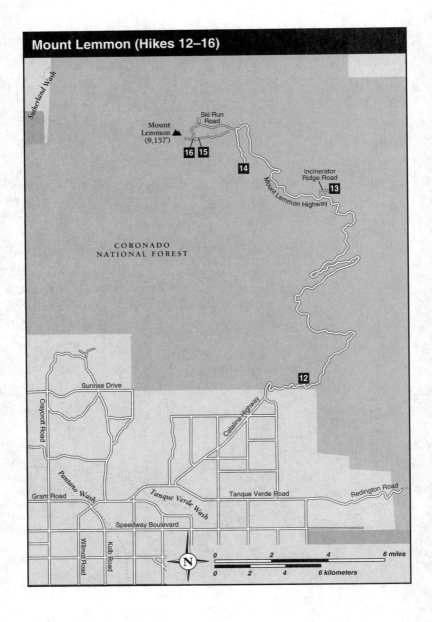

Mount Lemmon (Hikes 12–16)

Sutherland Wash

Ski Run Road

Mount Lemmon ▲ (9,157')

16 **15**

14

Incinerator Ridge Road **13**

Mount Lemmon Highway

CORONADO NATIONAL FOREST

Sunrise Drive

Craycroft Road

Catalina Highway

12

Pantano Wash

Grant Road

Tanque Verde Wash

Tanque Verde Road

Redington Road

Speedway Boulevard

Wilmot Road

Kolb Road

N

| 0 | 2 | 4 | 6 miles |
| 0 | 2 | 4 | 6 kilometers |

Mount Lemmon

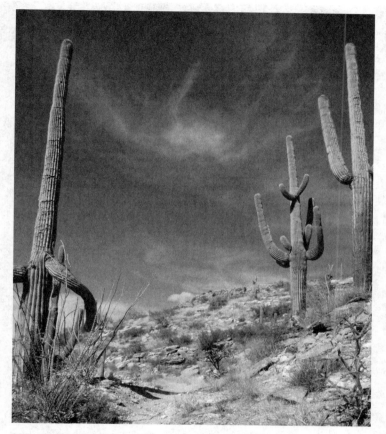

SAGUAROS FLANK THIS STRETCH OF THE BABAD DO'AG TRAIL.
(See next page.)

Babad Do'ag Trail

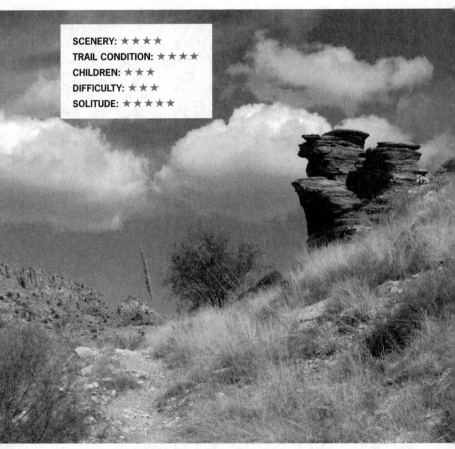

SCENERY: ★ ★ ★ ★
TRAIL CONDITION: ★ ★ ★ ★
CHILDREN: ★ ★ ★
DIFFICULTY: ★ ★ ★
SOLITUDE: ★ ★ ★ ★ ★

THE BABAD DO'AG TRAIL REACHES OAK WOODLANDS.

GPS TRAILHEAD COORDINATES: N32° 18.555' W110°43.240'

DISTANCE AND CONFIGURATION: 4-mile out-and-back

HIKING TIME: 2.5 hours

HIGHLIGHTS: Pretty waterfall after snowmelt or monsoon rains; changes in flora from saguaros to oaks; surprising view of Catalina Highway from ridge at trail end

ELEVATION: 3,568' at parking lot, 4,656' at trail's end

ACCESS: Open 24/7; free

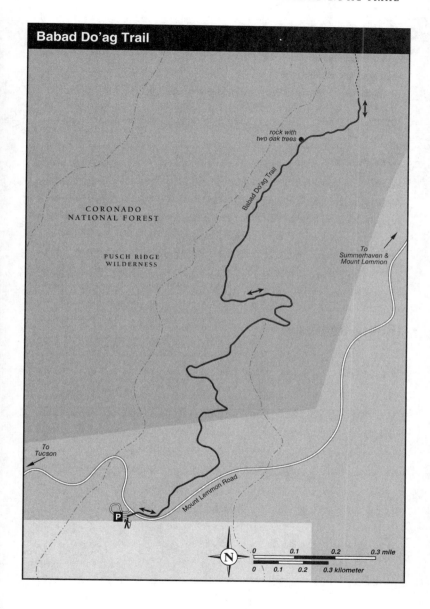

Babad Do'ag Trail

rock with
two oak trees

Babad Do'ag Trail

CORONADO
NATIONAL FOREST

PUSCH RIDGE
WILDERNESS

To
Summerhaven &
Mount Lemmon

To
Tucson

Mount Lemmon Road

P

| 0 | 0.1 | | 0.2 | 0.3 mile |

| 0 | 0.1 | 0.2 | 0.3 kilometer |

N

MAPS: Green Trails *Map 2886S–Santa Catalina Mountains*

FACILITIES: Parking for 17 vehicles. The Palisade Visitor Center is about 17 miles farther up Mount Lemmon.

WHEELCHAIR ACCESS: None

COMMENTS: Horses allowed but rarely encountered. Dogs must be leashed at all times. This elevation gets very hot in summer.

CONTACTS: Sabino Canyon Visitor Center, 520-749-8700, **www.fs.usda.gov/coronado**

Overview

This trail starts from near the first parking area on General Hitch-cock Highway, also known locally as Mount Lemmon Road. The trail climbs steadily but has no very steep sections, and the views of both the vegetation and the mountains are rewarding. The waterfall at the end is dry for most of the year; try to get there early on August mornings after the monsoons or in February and March during snowmelt to see water flowing.

Route Details

Start by driving to the scenic vista and parking area named Babad Do'ag, which means "Frog Mountain" in the Tohono O'odham language. Here, check out the panels identifying some of the mountains on the horizon before you walk out of the parking area and turn right (northeast). There is no sidewalk, so cross the road with care and walk up about 100 yards to a sign misspelled "Babat Duag"; this is Trail #705. Climb left from the road along an unclear trail for the first 50 yards—it's hard to follow, but cast around and you'll soon find a trail paralleling the road below. After another 200–300 yards, the trail swings sharply left away from the road to the northwest, following a normally dry little stream bed, and then becomes quite clear for the rest of the way.

You'll be treading on a mixed dirt, sand, and rock surface for which decent hiking footwear is recommended to avoid a twisted ankle. Around you, prickly pear cacti, ocotillos, and mesquite trees surround saguaros spread out on the hillside. This is almost the highest limit for saguaros, and as you rise above the 4,000-foot-elevation mark, you'll see the vegetation change into thickets of small oak trees surrounded by chaparral and grassland. It's remarkable to see this transition from saguaro forest to oak woodland, and this is one of the best trails from which to observe the transformation.

As you climb, you'll see a valley to your left and a ridge to your right. When you reach a rock where two oaks grow, the trail forks. The left fork is a social trail wandering off to explore the valley; the main trail climbs right (northeast). A few more minutes of hiking brings you to a saddle where you'll find a sign marking the end of the trail.

There are fine views from here. To the northwest, you'll see the waterfall at about the same elevation as the trail end, and there are unmarked social trails that will get you closer. To the east-northeast, the landscape drops steeply to the curves of Mount Lemmon Road as it hugs the slopes of Molino Canyon, beyond which are Agua Caliente Hill and the Rincon Mountains. To the east-southeast, social trails gain different views of Mount Lemmon Road, and far off to the south are the Santa Rita Mountains. It's a scenic spot to enjoy a snack before returning the way you came.

Nearby Attractions

Molino Basin Campground is reached by a turnoff from Catalina Highway, almost 3 miles beyond the Babad Do'ag parking area. It has 37 sites, drinking water, and vault toilets, but no hookups. It allows RVs or trailers up to 22 feet, charges $10 per night, and is open November–April. Most sites are first-come, first-served. Other campgrounds on the mountain are higher and are open in summer; this one is closed in summer because of the heat. More information: 877-444-6667, **recreation.gov**.

Directions

From central Tucson, take Broadway or Speedway Boulevard east to Wilmot Road. Turn left on Wilmot, which veers right at Pima Street and becomes Tanque Verde Road. Travel east on Tanque Verde for about 4 miles, then turn left on Catalina Highway, which veers northeast and goes straight almost 4.5 miles before reaching the Coronado National Forest boundary. This is Milepost 0 on what is locally known as Mount Lemmon Road (but which the U.S. Forest Service calls General Hitchcock Highway), a Sky Island Scenic Byway. Follow the highway almost 3 more miles to the Babad Do'ag scenic vista and parking area, on your right. Note that there are no gas stations on Catalina Highway or Mount Lemmon Road.

From I-10, coming from the southeast, take Exit 270/Kolb Road and follow it north for 10.5 miles to Tanque Verde Road. Turn right, drive 3.5 miles, and turn left on Catalina Highway.

From I-10, coming from the northwest, take Exit 256/Grant Road and head east. After 8.5 miles, turn left on Tanque Verde Road and drive 3.5 miles to Catalina Highway.

13

Incinerator Ridge Trail

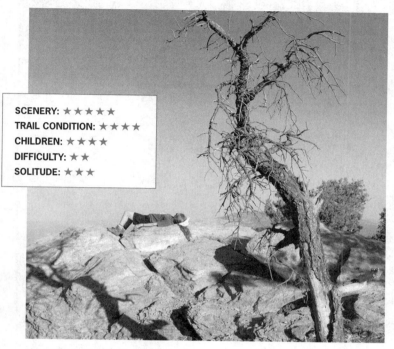

SCENERY: ★ ★ ★ ★ ★
TRAIL CONDITION: ★ ★ ★ ★
CHILDREN: ★ ★ ★ ★
DIFFICULTY: ★ ★
SOLITUDE: ★ ★ ★

RELAXING ON LEOPOLD POINT

GPS TRAILHEAD COORDINATES: N32° 24.700' W110° 42.326'

DISTANCE AND CONFIGURATION: 1.3-mile out-and-back

HIKING TIME: 1 hour

HIGHLIGHTS: Excellent views from a minor peak

ELEVATION: 8,000' at trailhead, 8,135' at high point

ACCESS: Open 24/7; free

MAPS: Green Trails *Map 2886S–Santa Catalina Mountains*

FACILITIES: Parking for 6 vehicles at trailhead

WHEELCHAIR ACCESS: None

COMMENTS: Horses and bicycles permitted but rarely seen; no dogs. Make alternate plans if the parking area is full. Mountain bikers find this one of the most difficult routes on Mount Lemmon.

CONTACTS: Sabino Canyon Visitor Center, 520-749-8700, **www.fs.usda.gov/coronado**

Incinerator Ridge Trail

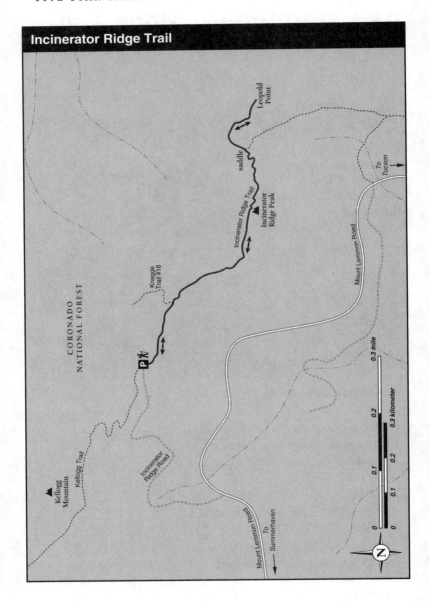

Overview

This short trail gives you a lot of bang for your shoe leather. There are excellent mountain, forest, and valley views all around (though you can't see Tucson), and the rock slabs at the end of the trail are great for resting and picnicking. The main drawback is the dirt access road leading to a diminutive parking area. Cars can get there with care but may find nowhere to park. In that case, if you return along the access road, you'll find a few spots where you can pull over and hike back up the road.

Route Details

Looking out over the north side of the parking area, you'll see a few twisted remains of what was once an incinerator—hence the name of this ridge. The trail leaves from the northeast corner of the parking area, signed "Incinerator Ridge Trail #18A." It climbs gently for 0.1 mile to the junction with Knagge Trail #18, which drops steeply to the left into the lowlands north of the Catalina Mountains. This trail is named after a family who mined in the area in the early 20th century and also provided pack-train services to the Summerhaven area before roads were available.

Stay on the Incinerator Ridge Trail as it continues flatly southeast. Looking to your right (south) through the pine trees, you'll catch glimpses of Catalina Highway below you. Soon you'll see a helicopter-landing pad to the south and, beyond it, Rose Canyon Lake, which at about 0.25 mile long is the largest lake in the Santa Catalina Mountains. Stocked with trout in summer, the lake has a campground nearby. Where the trail reaches the ridge, you can see the small communities of San Manuel and Mammoth in the San Pedro River valley to the northeast.

The trail begins to climb again and swings east as it reaches Incinerator Ridge Peak (8,135 feet) almost 0.4 mile from the trailhead. This is the highest point on the trail, but the best views are farther away, on the slightly lower peak directly east. The trail drops clearly into a saddle at about 7,960 feet elevation between these two peaks. Here, you'll find two trails, unsigned as of this writing. One drops to the right (southeast); this trail, completed in late 2012, goes to the San Pedro Vista lookout on Catalina Highway.

Our trail climbs left (north-northeast) into an area of large boulders. You'll round the left (north) side of Leopold Point, making your way through the boulders as you climb to the top of the peak. The high point is marked by a log stuck vertically into the summit rocks. Continue east about 100 feet to an inviting ledge with views in all directions, pull out a snack, and relax.

Leopold Point (8,050 feet) isn't marked on most maps—I found it on an obscure USGS map. It's probably named after writer, environmentalist, and forester Aldo Leopold (1887–1948), who worked for the U.S. Forest Service in the southwestern states, including two years stationed in Arizona.

The views here are superb in all directions. South is a precipitous cliff, Barnum Rock, about 0.4 mile away, and beyond to the southeast is Tucson, backed by the Santa Rita Mountains. East-northeast, back the way you came, has views of the radio towers on Mount Bigelow.

North are views into the San Pedro River valley. Bring a map and compass and enjoy picking out landmarks, then return the way you came.

Nearby Attractions

The **Palisade Visitor Center,** 0.4 mile farther along Catalina Highway, has information, maps, books, and a gift shop. It's usually open Thursday–Monday, 8 a.m.–4.30 p.m.

Rose Canyon Campground (877-444-6667, **recreation.gov**) is reached by a turnoff from Catalina Highway, 2.2 miles before Incinerator Ridge Road. With 74 sites, this is the largest campground on the mountain and has drinking water and vault toilets, but no hookups. **Spencer Canyon Campground** (520-749-8700, **www.fs.usda.gov /coronado**), reached by a turnoff 2.1 miles above Incinerator Ridge Road, has 62 sites and similar facilities. Both allow RVs or trailers up to 22 feet, charge $18 per night, and are open mid-April–late October. Most sites are first-come, first-served. For camping in winter, see Nearby Attractions for the previous hike.

Directions

Follow the directions for Hike 12, Babad Do'ag Trail (page 106), to reach Milepost 0 on Mount Lemmon Road (Catalina Highway). From Milepost 0, drive 19.3 miles to the poorly marked Incinerator Ridge Road, on your right. (If you reach the Palisade Visitor Center, you've driven 0.4 mile too far.) Incinerator Ridge Road, unpaved but passable for cars if you drive carefully, reaches the tiny parking turnaround after 0.5 mile.

14

Marshall Gulch Loop

SCENERY: ★ ★ ★ ★
TRAIL CONDITION: ★ ★ ★ ★
CHILDREN: ★ ★ ★ ★
DIFFICULTY: ★ ★ ★
SOLITUDE: ★ ★

MINI-WATERFALL IN MARSHALL GULCH

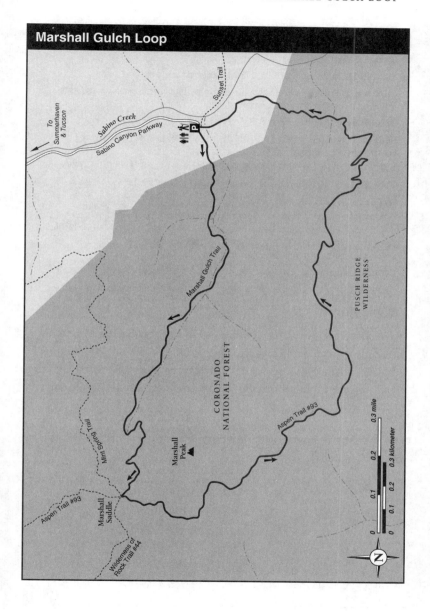

Marshall Gulch Loop

GPS TRAILHEAD COORDINATES: N32° 26.216' W110° 46.394'

DISTANCE AND CONFIGURATION: 3.6-mile loop, 2.4-mile out-and-back to Marshall Saddle

HIKING TIME: 2.25 hours for loop, 1.5 miles out-and-back to saddle

HIGHLIGHTS: Exploring one of Sabino Creek's highest tributaries; pine, oak, and aspen forests; cliff views; summer flowers; fall colors

ELEVATION: 7,460' at trailhead, 8,160' at high point

ACCESS: Open 24/7; parking $5/$10/$20 for day/week/year; all National Park Service annual passes accepted

MAPS: Green Trails *Map 2886S–Santa Catalina Mountains,* USFS *Pusch Ridge Wilderness*

FACILITIES: Pit toilets at trailhead; parking for about 18 cars (no trailers or RVs)

WHEELCHAIR ACCESS: Toilets only

COMMENTS: Horses allowed but rarely encountered. Dogs must be leashed at all times. If the parking area is full (most summer weekends), look for spaces along the road to the trailhead or in several small lots adjoining picnic areas along the last 0.5 mile of the road. The trail may be closed by snow in the winter.

CONTACTS: Sabino Canyon Visitor Center, 520-749-8700, **www.fs.usda.gov/coronado**

Overview

This is a very popular loop hike for Tucsonans looking to beat the summer heat. Combined with a picnic lunch or a visit to a Summerhaven restaurant (see Nearby Attractions), this hike completes a relaxing day in the mountains. Going counterclockwise, as described here, the trail follows an evergreen-forested stream and later emerges to yield rocky vistas, followed by a saddle and aspen groves. Other hikers may prefer the clockwise route, which starts off more steeply.

Route Details

At the north end of the parking area, to the right of the toilets, look for a sign indicating Marshall Gulch Trail #3 and a narrow trail zigzagging right and up into the trees. After a couple of brief switchbacks, the trail straightens and climbs west through an evergreen forest of ponderosa pine and Douglas-fir, mixed with oaks and madrones. Down below to your left, the terrain drops to Marshall Gulch, a tributary of Sabino Creek (which ends up in Sabino Canyon). The trail stays high for less than 0.5 mile before dropping and easily crossing the narrow stream.

Almost immediately after you make your way across the stream, you'll reach a T-junction, where you turn right. (Left takes you back to the parking lot, following the stream bed and easily crossing it again for a loop of less than a mile.)

The trail climbs very gently, with the stream teasing you to your right. There's water in it almost all year long. Take your time, enjoy the sounds of nature, and maybe cool your feet. Before you know it, you'll be crossing the stream again, from left to right, climbing west-northwest into the forest. After several hundred yards of hiking, you might notice a small weather station on the right side of the trail with rain gauges measuring rainfall variability in the Santa Catalina Mountains. About 100 yards farther, the trail crosses the stream a final time, from right to left.

Continue climbing steadily through ferns surrounding a mix of burned and living pines. High to the northwest on the aptly named Radio Ridge, which leads up to Mount Lemmon, you'll see several communication towers. A final push up a rocky trail with views of granite cliffs and outcrops brings you to Marshall Saddle (7,920 feet), where signs point out the five trails that meet at this point. (If you hike the Wilderness of Rock Loop, page 128, you'll again reach this significant hiking crossroads.)

While resting at the saddle, look a few degrees north of west to spy Lemmon Rock Lookout, a U.S. Forest Service fire lookout perched atop a cliff; you can visit it on the Meadow Trail (see next hike). Hikers on the Arizona National Scenic Trail will discover that Marshall Gulch is a tiny section of the 800-mile trail that crosses the entire state, from Mexico to the Utah state line.

From Marshall Saddle, you can return the way you came, making an out-and-back hike of 2.4 miles, or turn left, heading south on signed Aspen Trail #93, to make the full loop. This is the area in which the devastating 2003 Aspen Fire started, and you can see remnants of the destruction mixed in with more than a decade of recovery. During

AFTERNOON MIST ON THE ASPEN TRAIL

late summer, in July and August, alpine wildflowers are prolific in this section. October is an excellent month to enjoy fall foliage.

The Aspen Trail climbs very gently, then flattens after it leaves Marshall Saddle. After several hundred yards, the trail swings southeast and then east as it contours around Marshall Peak (about 8,300 feet) to the left of the trail. There is no path to the elongated, wooded summit, though adventurous hikers could bushwhack up there. Most hikers look toward the right of the trail, where they can glimpse Tucson to the south and southwest through the trees. Look for unsigned side trails leaving the Aspen Trail to the right to gain better views of Tucson.

Continuing east on the Aspen Trail, you'll climb to the high point of the loop, although it's hard to tell which is the highest point as the trail undulates through the forest. The last mile swings around to the north and drops, sometimes steeply, with views of the cliffs of the uppermost reaches of Sabino Canyon to the right; again, unsigned short side trails will give better views. As you hike through this last section, look around for quartz and mica specks, which glisten on a sunny day.

The trail tumbles down to the Marshall Gulch parking area. If you prefer hiking the trail clockwise, in reverse of this description, you'll find a sign for Aspen Trail #93 at the south end of the parking area, from which it climbs steeply to the south before swinging around to the west.

Nearby Attractions

About a mile before the trailhead, Sabino Canyon Parkway, the approach road, passes through the village of **Summerhaven**. Almost half of the village was destroyed in the summer of 2003, when about 340 homes and businesses burned during the disastrous Aspen Fire. Summerhaven continues to recover and offers a couple of eateries and a village store–cum–gift shop, but no gas station.

South of the village, several parking lots adjoin the uppermost reaches of Sabino Creek and provide access to many cool, shady picnic areas with tables and barbecue grills. These parking lots serve as overflow parking for the nearby Marshall Gulch/Aspen trailhead. The road and parking areas close during winter snows.

Directions

Follow the directions for Hike 12, Babad Do'ag Trail (page 106), to reach Milepost 0 on Mount Lemmon Road (Catalina Highway). From Milepost 0, drive about 25 miles to the village of Summerhaven and continue another mile to the Marshall Gulch trailhead. Note that there is no gas in Summerhaven, so make sure you've left Tucson with several gallons in your tank.

HIKERS ON THE MARSHALL GULCH TRAIL

15

Meadow Trail Loop

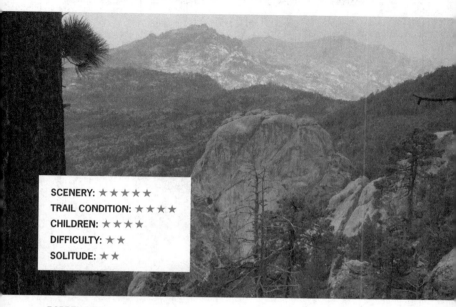

SCENERY: ★ ★ ★ ★ ★
TRAIL CONDITION: ★ ★ ★ ★
CHILDREN: ★ ★ ★ ★
DIFFICULTY: ★ ★
SOLITUDE: ★ ★

RAPPEL ROCK

GPS TRAILHEAD COORDINATES: N32° 26.416' W110° 47.151'

DISTANCE AND CONFIGURATION: 1.6-mile loop, 2.1 miles with side trip to lookout

HIKING TIME: 1-hour loop, 1.5 hours with side trip

HIGHLIGHTS: Fine views of Tucson; exceptional views from lookout; pretty meadows surrounded by coniferous forest

ELEVATION: 9,100' at trailhead, 8,800' at low point

ACCESS: Open 24/7; parking $5/$10/$20 for day/week/year; all National Park Service annual passes accepted

MAPS: Green Trails *Map 2886S–Santa Catalina Mountains*, USFS *Pusch Ridge Wilderness*

FACILITIES: Pit toilets at trailhead; parking for about 20 cars (no trailers or RVs)

WHEELCHAIR ACCESS: Toilets only

COMMENTS: Horses allowed but rarely encountered. Dogs must be leashed at all times. If the parking area is full, look for spaces along the road to the trailhead or in the unmarked parking area near the top of the ski area, about 0.2 mile back along the road on the south side. The trail and road may be closed by snow in the winter—but it's a short winter in southern Arizona!

CONTACTS: Sabino Canyon Visitor Center, 520-749-8700, **www.fs.usda.gov/coronado**

Meadow Trail Loop

0.3 mile
0.3 kilometer

To Catalina Highway

Ski Valley Road

Mount Lemmon (9,157')

Steward Observatory

Mount Lemmon Trail

Lemmon Rock Fire Lookout

Lemmon Rock Lookout Trail

Meadow Trail

Mount Lemmon Trail

CORONADO NATIONAL FOREST

Overview

This lovely loop takes you through alpine meadows and conifer forests before reaching views of Tucson. The first section is flat and suitable for introducing pre-kindergarten youngsters to the high country. A gentle 300-foot descent loops around to a side trail that heads to a fire lookout with extensive views of southern Arizona—this view is the only reason the hike gets five stars for scenery. The final return is a slightly steep challenge for the young ones in your party.

Route Details

At the parking area, you'll find a map board and a sign for Mount Lemmon Trail #5. Take this trail, which skirts around the chain-link fence surrounding electrical power equipment, before striking out west-southwest through the pines. After about 0.2 mile you'll reach a signed trail fork where you take the right (west-northwest) branch, labeled "Meadow Trail #5A." This short side trail, which will return to the Mount Lemmon Trail after 0.8 mile, gives this hike its name.

Through the trees to your right (north), you'll glimpse buildings belonging to the University of Arizona astronomy observatory (see

Nearby Attractions). The trail traverses a mix of ferns, bracken, and living and dead conifers—a legacy of the devastating Aspen Fire of 2003. As the trail's name suggests, meadows are crossed, and you have intermittent views of Tucson to the south. The trail is clear and rather rocky.

About 0.5 mile from the parking lot, the trail swings left (southwest), away from the university buildings, and continues fairly flatly for a few hundred yards through meadows and pine forests. Then it eases into a gentle descent, which steepens into an easy zigzag on an earthen trail through continuing pines.

You reach the halfway point of the loop when the Meadow Trail rejoins the Mount Lemmon Trail at a signed intersection. There are good views to the south, with Thimble Peak and Sabino Canyon's Phoneline Trail clearly visible at 162° to the southeast. At this junction, near the low point of the trail, turn left (east-northeast, then east) along the Mount Lemmon Trail, which roughly follows the 8,800-foot contour line.

You'll enjoy views of the Tucson valley to your right and gently begin to climb until you reach a signed turn for the Lemmon Rock Lookout Trail #12 to the right (south-southeast). Here, you can continue on Mount Lemmon Trail to the northeast and back to the parking area, or you can head south on the recommended side trip to the Lemmon Rock Lookout.

The Lemmon Rock Lookout Trail descends through the pine forest and continues down to the Wilderness of Rock (see page 128). Wander down just a few hundred yards to the turnoff to the lookout on your left, then climb to the lookout tower itself. There has been a lookout here since 1913, and the current tower is open to visitors during the dry summer fire season, when it is occupied around the clock by a U.S. Forest Service firefighter who spends the entire summer in the cramped but totally scenic quarters. When Audrey and I visited, we were warmly welcomed by firefighter Dave Medford and his dog, Gus.

Dave pointed out all the landmarks and mountain ranges visible from his lookout, explaining the southern-Arizona weather patterns that he can see unfolding above, below, and around him. Gus enjoyed getting a head rub until he was back on duty, with a friendly bark to alert us to the arrival of the next visitors.

If you're here outside of the fire season, the views from the rock upon which the lookout tower is built are almost as great as from the tower itself. Looking west, you'll see three nearby outcrops that are favored by rock climbers. The one on the left is Rappel Rock, the middle one is Fortress Rock, and the series of slabs to the right are The Ravens. Way off to the south and southwest, the Tucson valley spreads out before you, surrounded in the distance by the Tucson, Santa Rita, and Rincon Mountains. It's a splendid survey of almost everywhere in this book.

Back on the Mount Lemmon Trail, you'll climb northeast on the steepest part of the loop. This is where the youngest members of your group might want a shoulder ride. It's wide and rocky until you reach the fork with the Meadow Trail. Turn right here to return to the trailhead.

Nearby Attractions

To the right of the entrance of the parking area is a sign for the **Mount Lemmon Sky Center** (520-626-8122, **skycenter.arizona.edu**). Part of the University of Arizona's Steward Observatory, it can be visited most nights on 5-hour guided tours, with opportunities for using large telescopes to view astronomical objects. Guided by enthusiastic professional astronomers, tours are limited to 20 people and cost $60 (discounts available). Reservations are recommended.

Directions

Follow the directions for Hike 12, Babad Do'ag Trail (page 106), to reach Milepost 0 on Mount Lemmon Road (Catalina Highway). From Milepost 0, drive 24.6 miles to the Ski Valley turnoff, to the right just before the village of Summerhaven. After about 2 miles, you'll pass through Mt. Lemmon Ski Valley and continue about 1.8 steep, curving miles to the trailhead. This last section is usually closed in winter.

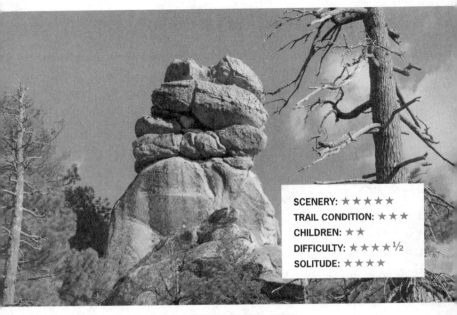

SCENERY: ★ ★ ★ ★
TRAIL CONDITION: ★ ★ ★
CHILDREN: ★ ★
DIFFICULTY: ★ ★ ★ ★ ½
SOLITUDE: ★ ★ ★ ★

ONE OF THE WILDERNESS'S MANY ROCK FORMATIONS

GPS TRAILHEAD COORDINATES: N32° 26.452' W110° 47.023'

DISTANCE AND CONFIGURATION: 5.9-mile downward loop

HIKING TIME: 4.25 hours

HIGHLIGHTS: Mount Lemmon Rock Lookout, views of precipices (sometimes with rock-climbers), rock formations, late-summer flowers

ELEVATION: 9,040' at trailhead, 7,200' at low point

ACCESS: 24/7 all year but limited or closed in winter depending on weather or snow conditions; parking $5/$10/$20 for day/week/year; all National Park Service annual passes accepted

MAPS: Green Trails *Map 2886S–Santa Catalina Mountains*, USFS *Pusch Ridge Wilderness*

FACILITIES: Pit toilets about 0.2 mile from trailhead; parking for about 15 cars (no trailers or RVs)

WHEELCHAIR ACCESS: None

COMMENTS: Horses allowed but rarely encountered. Dogs must be leashed at all times. If the parking area is full, look for spaces along the road beyond the parking area or in the second parking area, about 0.2 mile farther along the road.

CONTACTS: Sabino Canyon Visitor Center, 520-749-8700, **www.fs.usda.gov/coronado**

Wilderness of Rock Loop

Mount Lemmon (9,157')

Ski Valley Road

Ski Valley Road

To Catalina Highway

chairlift

Meadow Trail

Mount Lemmon Trail

Lemmon Rock Fire Lookout

Lemmon Rock Lookout Trail

Aspen Trail #93

Marshall Saddle

Mint Spring Trail

Marshall Gulch Trail

Aspen Trail #93

CORONADO
NATIONAL FOREST

PUSCH RIDGE
WILDERNESS

Wilderness of Rock Trail #44

N

0   0.1   0.2   0.3 mile
0   0.1 0.2 0.3 kilometer

Overview

This cool, high hike is a great way to spend a summer day away from Tucson's heat. You'll start just below the summit of Mount Lemmon and descend steeply almost 2,000 feet, past rock formations and through pine forests. The Wilderness of Rock is an area of mainly granite boulders and cliffs forming a wide band around the south side of the higher sections of Mount Lemmon. This loop enters the eastern part of the wilderness and exits via the popular Marshall Gulch saddle and up to the top of Mt. Lemmon Ski Valley, Tucson's backyard ski area.

Route Details

From the unsigned, unpaved parking area on the left side of the road, at the top of the ski area, look for a trail paralleling the left side of the road, going west-southwest and offering great views of the Tucson valley to your left. In just under 0.2 mile you'll arrive at the parking area for the Meadow Trail (see page 123), where you can also park, but this lot is often full in summer.

Find a map board and a sign for Mount Lemmon Trail #5. Take this trail, which skirts around the chain-link fence surrounding electrical power equipment, before striking out west-southwest through the pines. After about 0.2 mile you'll reach a signed trail fork—take the left branch, heading generally southwest and downhill for 0.4 mile to the beginning of Lemmon Rock Lookout Trail #12. A sign indicates it to your left.

Descend south on the Lemmon Rock Lookout Trail for about 0.2 mile to where the trail makes a sharp right hairpin turn. (At this point, if you continue straight for about 100 yards, you can visit the fire lookout described in the previous hike.) The Lemmon Rock Lookout Trail now starts descending in earnest, and a sign informs you that you're entering the Santa Catalina Natural Area. If you're here in August—which is late spring at these elevations—you'll see many wildflowers along the trail. To the west are fine views of the huge slabs of Ravens Rock and, below them, the popular rock-climbing outcrop appropriately named Rappel Rock. If you're lucky, you'll catch sight of ant-sized climbers silhouetted against the sky.

The trail does nothing but switchback down past these sights, and after about a mile of descent it crosses a small creek bed, which may have water in it during all but the driest months of early summer. Beyond, the rough, loose, rocky trail continues its inexorable descent with more switchbacks. You'll have been walking through mixed pine–oak woodland, with both living and burned trees—it's amazing how some survived and others were destroyed by the Aspen Fire. As you get lower, you'll start seeing some of the oddly shaped boulders that give the Wilderness of Rock its name.

Eventually, some 2.6 miles from the trailhead, you'll reach a T-junction that's the lowest point of the trail. Here, turn hard left onto Wilderness of Rock Trail #44. There is a place to camp, but if you're so inclined, you'll find better spots with rough fire rings 100 yards up the trail. A small stream paralleling this trail might have water in spring after snowmelt and in late summer after the monsoons, and trickles in other months. The creek usually dries out in mid-summer.

Now the trail climbs steadily to the east and northeast, crossing the stream numerous times in the first mile of the fairly gentle climb. As you get higher, keep your eyes open to the left for views of the Lemmon Rock Lookout and the towers of Radio Ridge. About 1.7 miles and 700 feet above the Wilderness of Rock trail junction, you reach the busy Marshall Saddle, also reached via the Marshall Gulch Loop (see page 116) from the other side.

Here, turn left (north) onto the signed Aspen Trail #93. This becomes a ridge trail, with views to the right (east) of burned trees and views to the left of surviving forest. Also to the right, on the skyline, you'll see the University of Arizona observatories. Aspen Trail becomes increasingly steep as it climbs north and then northwest toward Radio Ridge. It's a 1.3-mile climb to the intersection with Aspen Draw Trail #423, where you turn left onto a dirt road, passing the top of the Ski Valley chairlift, electric pylons, and radio towers, until you reach the road and your car, 0.2 mile past the ski area.

Nearby Attractions

In mid-winter, you might find the trail closed or impassable because of snow. Instead, take the opportunity of a few runs at **Mt. Lemmon Ski Valley** (520-576-1321, **skithelemmon.com**), the southernmost ski area in the United States. Admittedly, the one good chairlift provides access to just 22 shortish runs, but it's fun and, by skiing standards, not expensive ($40 all-day admission for adults; various discounts available). The season, limited by snowfall, varies from a couple of weeks to a couple of months—check the website. During the summer, the lift becomes a Sky Ride ($9 for adults), with round-trip views in all directions. In October, Ski Valley holds an Oktoberfest, with oompah music, German food and beer, and golden fall views.

Directions

See previous hike.

CLIMBER ON RAPPEL ROCK

Santa Catalina Foothills (Hikes 17–23)

Santa Catalina Foothills

ROCK FORMATIONS IN THE UPPER REACHES OF FINGER ROCK CANYON
(see Hike 19, page 147)

Catalina State Park:
Nature and Birding Loops

SCENERY: ★ ★ ★ ★
TRAIL CONDITION: ★ ★ ★ ★ ★
CHILDREN: ★ ★ ★ ★
DIFFICULTY: ★ ★
SOLITUDE: ★ ★

HORSES ARE PROHIBITED ON THE BIRDING TRAIL, BUT LIZARDS ARE WELCOME.

GPS TRAILHEAD COORDINATES: N32° 25.581' W110° 54.454'

DISTANCE AND CONFIGURATION: 2-mile figure-eight

HIKING TIME: 1 hour or, for birders, as long as you want

HIGHLIGHTS: Great views of Pusch Ridge, interpretive signs, fun introduction to the Arizona–Sonora desert

ELEVATION: 2,720' at trailhead, 2,805' at high point

ACCESS: Trail open 24/7; $7 per carload (1–4 passengers), $3 per pedestrian or bicyclist

MAPS: Green Trails *Map 2886S–Santa Catalina Mountains,* USFS *Pusch Ridge Wilderness;* free sketch map at visitor center

FACILITIES: Ranger station and gift shop, open 8 a.m.–5 p.m.; campground with showers and flush toilets; drinking water; picnic areas; equestrian center; large parking area at trailhead with seasonal gift shop and pit toilets

Catalina State Park: Nature and Birding Loops

WHEELCHAIR ACCESS: For developed areas; none for trails

COMMENTS: Leashed pets and mountain bikes allowed

CONTACTS: Catalina State Park, 520-628-5798, **azstateparks.com/parks/cata**

Overview

This figure-eight trail combines two 1-mile-long loop trails that both leave from Catalina State Park's main trailhead, so you can just do one if you're pressed for time. Both are trails for slow hiking, reading the interpretive signs, and perhaps introducing small children to the wonders of the Arizona-Sonora desert. There are a few steepish sections, but they don't last long. The mountain views are a bonus!

Route Details

From the north end of the parking area, to your left as you face the road, walk about 100 yards to a small traffic circle that is the end of the road and has three trailheads. Ignoring the main Romero Canyon Trailhead, go to the northernmost part of the traffic circle and a Nature Trail sign. Within 100 yards, another sign shows six possible trails—again, follow the Nature Trail sign.

Now you'll climb steeply but briefly up a wide trail of mixed rocks and sand to the first of numerous interpretive signs on this hike. Looking right (south and southeast), you'll enjoy views of Sutherland Wash below and the mountains of Pusch Ridge on the close horizon above. The sheer-sided, flat-topped, blocky peak to the south is the unimaginatively named Table Mountain. Roughly east, you'll see Romero Canyon (see page 141).

After another 5 minutes of easy climbing, you'll reach a fork for the Nature Trail Loop. It doesn't much matter which way you walk it; I describe it going left (west). There are frequent informative signs—I like the cement slabs with animal footprints, which remind me of movie stars' handprints on the Hollywood Walk of Fame. Javelinas, coyotes, and roadrunners are certainly the stars of the southwestern deserts.

Benches are intermittently placed for hikers to rest and to enjoy the view. One of the benches is dedicated to Gale W. Monson (1912–2012) and his wife, Sarah. Considered a father of Arizonan field ornithology, Monson was one of the authors of the first annotated checklist of Arizona birds. This is as good a place as any to identify your first cactus wren.

Continue around this 1-mile loop and return to the Nature Trail Loop sign; then descend to the sign showing six trails, mentioned earlier. Here, turn left (east) toward the Birding Trail. You'll soon have a couple of choices, either skirting around the side of the road to the southeast or taking a trail to the southeast, but either way you'll quickly get to the Romero Canyon Trail and turn south, crossing Sutherland Wash. This is normally dry or has an easily negotiated shallow flow of water. Rarely, a minor wade may be necessary.

South of Sutherland Wash, you'll almost immediately see a sign for the Birding Trail to the right. The wide trail, like most of the lower trails in this area, meanders through a mesquite bosque (woodland), and you can appreciate how thorny the mesquite tree is. Its bean-like pods bear seeds that were ground into flour to provide southwestern Native Americans with sustenance. Nowadays, you're most likely to encounter the gastronomy of mesquite as a natural flavor of bee honey or smoked meat.

After about 0.2 mile the trail reaches the Birding Trail Loop, described here going left (south), though you can go either way. Barely 0.1 mile beyond, the trail crosses the usually dry Montrose Wash and begins to climb steps fashioned from railroad ties to the top of a small mesa. Frequent signs describe the natural history of the area; there are also benches to rest on, and fine Pusch Ridge views.

The best time for photographs of sunlight on Pusch Ridge is in the 2 hours before sunset, which coincides with one of the two best times for birding and animal-watching (the other is the hours after sunrise). After strolling around the small mesa, walk down another set of stairs, recross Montrose Wash, and rejoin the trail, heading left (north) back to the parking area.

Nearby Attractions

Another worthwhile loop is the informatively signed **Romero Ruins Interpretive Trail,** an easy 0.75-mile walk that passes a saguaro with more than 30 arms, and loops through the indistinct foundations of a small Hohokam village and the more obvious remnants of the Romero ranch. The trail leaves from the right side of the park road, about halfway between the entrance and the trailhead described earlier. A picnic area across the road provides parking.

Two miles north of the park, the nonprofit **Western National Parks Association** (12880 N. Vistoso Village Dr., Oro Valley; 520-622-6014, **wnpa.org**) sells Tucson's widest variety of outdoor books, along with field guides, maps, music, hiking equipment, and authentic Native American crafts and jewelry. Hours are Monday–Saturday, 9:30 a.m.–5 p.m. They also offer free lectures and sell workshops and tours. Reach the store by turning north from Catalina State Park on Oracle Road, driving 1.7 miles to Rancho Vistoso Boulevard, turning left (west), and driving 0.3 mile to Innovation Park Drive. Turn left here and drive 0.25 mile; the store is on your left.

See the next hike for more nearby attractions.

Directions

See next hike.

18

Catalina State Park:
Romero Canyon Trail to Romero Pools

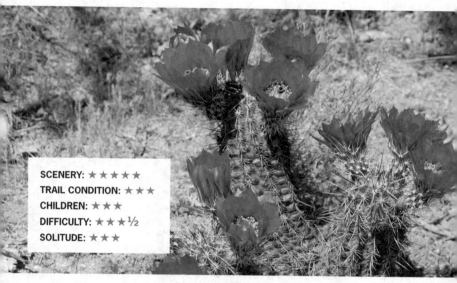

SCENERY: ★ ★ ★ ★ ★
TRAIL CONDITION: ★ ★ ★
CHILDREN: ★ ★ ★
DIFFICULTY: ★ ★ ★ ½
SOLITUDE: ★ ★ ★

HEDGEHOG CACTUS BLOOMS BRILLIANTLY IN APRIL AND MAY.

GPS TRAILHEAD COORDINATES: N32° 25.532' W110°54.465'

DISTANCE AND CONFIGURATION: 5.6-mile out-and-back, 6.7-mile loop via Canyon Loop Trail

HIKING TIME: 4 hours

HIGHLIGHTS: Gorgeous high-desert flora; mountain and desert views; pools to cool your feet

ELEVATION: 2,720' at trailhead, 3,680' at high point, 3,600' at pools

ACCESS: Open 24/7; $7 per carload (1–4 passengers); $3 per pedestrian or bicyclist

MAPS: Green Trails *Map 2886S–Santa Catalina Mountains*, USFS *Pusch Ridge Wilderness*; free sketch map at visitor center

FACILITIES: Ranger station and gift shop, open 8 a.m.–5 p.m.; campground with showers and flush toilets; drinking water; picnic areas; equestrian center; large parking area at trailhead with seasonal gift shop and pit toilets

WHEELCHAIR ACCESS: For developed areas; none for trails

COMMENTS: The first 1.25 miles of the trail are in Catalina State Park, where leashed pets, horses, and mountain bikes are allowed. The rest of the trail is in Coronado National Forest, where pets and bikes are prohibited.

CONTACTS: Catalina State Park, 520-628-5798, **azstateparks.com/parks/cata;** Coronado National Forest, 520-749-8700, **www.fs.usda.gov/coronado**

Catalina State Park: Romero Canyon Trail to Romero Pools

Overview

This rocky trail follows yet another of the many gorgeous canyons climbing into the Catalinas. Great mountain views and high desert flora characterize the hike, and wildlife ranging from skunks to deer has been reported, although most people will see only lizards and birds. The seasonal Romero Pools invite exploration and are a good turnaround point, although the trail continues high into the Catalinas, connecting with trails that lead to Mount Lemmon, Sabino Canyon, and other landmarks.

Route Details

The canyon is named after the Romero family, who were ranchers in the area in the mid-to-late 19th century. Records vary, but Francisco Romero seems to have been the first settler here, and ruins of his house can be seen on the 0.75-mile Romero Ruins Interpretive Trail, elsewhere in the park.

The Romero Canyon Trail leaves south from the trailhead at the northeast end of the main park road. (There are three trailheads within 100 yards of one another—this is the main one, and well signed).

Almost immediately you'll cross the wide and usually sandy Sutherland Wash, although you may need to negotiate some water after heavy rain. Beyond the wash, at a trail signpost, turn left (northeast) to climb a sandy trail that soon swings east and reaches another signed junction, 0.6 mile from the trailhead—here, take the right fork. (Going left, on the Canyon Loop Trail, is a 2.3-mile loop back to the trailhead and is an alternate return from the Romero Pools hike, described below.)

The trail continues through a mesquite bosque and, 0.5 mile from the previous junction, reaches the signed turnoff to Montrose Pools. (You can take a brief side trip south, to the right, to a bench overlooking the seasonal pools in a steep canyon below. A rough trail switchbacks down to the pools.) The Romero Canyon Trail turns left (east) and becomes much narrower as it climbs steps made with railroad ties to prevent erosion. Soon after the Montrose Pools junction, a sign indicates that you are entering Coronado National Forest.

OCOTILLO FLOWERS ON ROMERO CANYON TRAIL

This area has gorgeously varied high desert flora: In April and May, ocotillos bloom reddish-orange, prickly pears boast yellow flowers, and hedgehog cacti present lilac-colored bouquets. Agaves, yuccas, and saguaros wait to enter the display in late May and June.

Eventually the trail flattens, and on your left you'll see some strange rocks that look like large chunks of dirt with fist-sized rocks embedded in them. The trail contours to the south for a few hundred yards and then climbs east again, through occasional narrow rocky passages and past ocotillos. You'll eventually catch sight of Romero Canyon to your left, but don't be tempted to descend if you see water. Follow the clear main trail until it reaches a minor saddle and then drops a few hundred yards to the pools.

Here, the trail crosses the water (except in dry months) and continues climbing 4.4 miles to Romero Pass, 2,400 feet above you. Most hikers stop to explore the pools, which stretch out for several hundred yards north and east of the crossing. Flattish areas to the northeast can make adequate wilderness campsites. The pools are seasonal, although some of the deeper, more sheltered ones almost always have a little water. After heavy rains you'll see waterfalls. At all times step carefully, because the rocks are slick with algae and you can easily take a tumble.

Return the way you came until you reach the signed right turn for the **Canyon Loop Trail.** Here, you can continue 0.6 mile to return to the trailhead, or you can turn right and hike 1.7 miles to enjoy the alternate longer (but easy and scenic) return route. This heads east and northeast through the mesquite bosque until a hairpin bend takes you suddenly north and west to two benches, where you can rest and enjoy superb views of the western Catalinas. Just beyond the benches, the trail forks—the left fork is for horses, and the right fork takes hikers down a curving flight of stairs into the canyon bottom.

Head west and then swing north, following the left bank of a seasonal creek for several hundred yards until a crossing, 0.9 mile from where you entered the Canyon Loop Trail. By this point the creek is more likely to be dry, depending on the season. Immediately past the crossing, a sign indicates the Sutherland Trail to the right, while the Canyon Loop Trail goes straight ahead. The well-signed trail swings west and then south, crossing the increasingly dry creek a few times. To the south and southwest are impressive views of the blocky mountains forming Pusch Ridge, the most obvious of which are the massive cliffs of Table Mountain.

Near the end of the route, the trail intersects the Birding and Nature Trails. The road is 20 yards beyond, and the parking area and Romero Canyon Trailhead are another 100 yards along the road.

Nearby Attractions

Catalina State Park has a very comfortable campground with flush toilets and hot showers. All sites have picnic tables and barbecue grills, but ground fires are prohibited. Drinking-water faucets are scattered frequently throughout. Nightly rates during the high season (January 1–March 31) are $20 for 25 nonelectric (tent) sites and $25 or $30 for 99 electric sites. During the hotter months, the rates are $5 less. Reservations, recommended in the high season, can be made online at **azstateparks.com/parks/cata** or by calling 520-586-2283. A nonrefundable $5 reservation fee applies.

See the previous hike for other nearby attractions.

Directions

Take Oracle Road (AZ 77), Tucson's major road going north from the west side of town, to Catalina State Park: From the intersection of Oracle and Grant Roads, drive north on Oracle to enter the town of Oro Valley and reach the entrance to Catalina State Park, on the right about 12.3 miles north of Grant Road. Turn right into the park, passing the ranger station after 0.4 mile—if the station is closed, use the self-pay ticket booth. Continue northeast about 2 more miles on a paved road to the trailhead, at the end of the road. There is ample parking and a restroom.

19

Finger Rock Trail to Mount Kimball

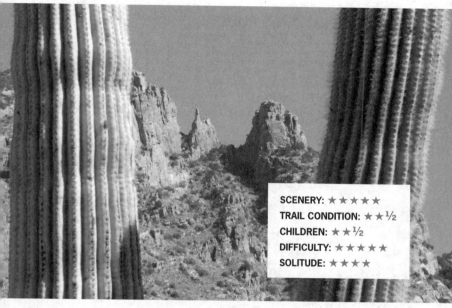

SCENERY: ★ ★ ★ ★ ★
TRAIL CONDITION: ★ ★ ½
CHILDREN: ★ ★ ½
DIFFICULTY: ★ ★ ★ ★ ★
SOLITUDE: ★ ★ ★ ★

FINGER ROCK VIEWED THROUGH THE ARMS OF A SAGUARO

GPS TRAILHEAD COORDINATES: N32° 20.215' W110° 54.600'

DISTANCE AND CONFIGURATION: 10.2-mile out-and-back

HIKING TIME: 8.5 hours

HIGHLIGHTS: Fabulous views of iconic Finger Rock; saguaro forest; bagging a peak with superb vistas

ELEVATION: 3,100' at trailhead, 7,258' at Mount Kimball

ACCESS: Trail open 24/7, parking lot open during daylight hours; free

MAPS: Green Trails *Map 2886S–Santa Catalina Mountains*, USFS *Pusch Ridge Wilderness*, USGS *Tucson North*

FACILITIES: Parking lot for 30 cars (no large vehicles) fills early on weekends; if it's full, overflow parking is available 0.2 mile back along Alvernon Way on gravel roadsides.

WHEELCHAIR ACCESS: None

COMMENTS: Dogs prohibited; no water available

CONTACTS: Coronado National Forest, 520-749-8700, **www.fs.usda.gov/coronado**

Finger Rock Trail to Mount Kimball

Overview

Finger Rock is a major landmark on Tucson's mountainous northern horizon. This steep, difficult, but clear trail climbs Finger Rock Canyon almost a vertical mile up into the Catalinas, never getting close to the pinnacle it's named after. Instead, it continues much higher, reaching a satisfying but uncomplicated summit from which you can see everything north of Tucson (but not the city itself). You'll enjoy climbing through changing ecosystems, from stands of saguaro to a pine forest.

Route Details

Start from the Richard "Dick" McKee Trailhead, at the north end of Alvernon Way about 100 yards from the parking lot. The trailhead's name honors Richard McKee, a conservationist and member of the Pima County Attorney's Environmental Enforcement Unit, who died in 1999 at age 43 from complications of leukemia. The Finger Rock Trail was one of his favorite hikes in the Catalinas.

The trailhead, shared with the Pontatoc Ridge Trail (see page 164), features informative notices about the bighorn mountain sheep herd that roam the area. They died out in the 1990s, and a herd of 30 bighorns from Yuma was reintroduced here in November 2013. Two very short, fairly steep switchbacks bring you to a signed trail fork where Finger Rock Trail #42 goes north. The trail, nearly flat to begin with, provides great views of the saguaro-forested lowlands, the digit-in-the-air Finger Rock, and the pine-forested mound of Mount Kimball to the right of the rock.

After about a mile of easy hiking with a gentle ascent, you'll notice a couple of large, green aspen trees to your left, indicating that there is indeed some water, some of the time, in Finger Rock Canyon. Maps mark a spring here. In this greener area, an unsigned trail, blocked with a row of stones, goes down to the left to explore the water, but the Finger Rock Trail begins to climb steeply to the right.

As you climb, you'll enjoy watching the canyon open to your left into a gorgeous bowl full of saguaros, with a lovely tan-colored wall rising vertically for about 500 feet on the opposite side of your trail. If you're here in spring, you'll see plenty of wildflowers along the trail. The trail is clear but quite difficult, with some leg-stretching steps, loose rocks, and awkwardly placed spiny plants of all kinds, often in rather exposed areas, so pay attention.

Eventually, you start climbing above the highest saguaros and lose sight of Finger Rock. The flora changes into pine–oak woodlands and—yay!—the trail actually becomes flat for a relaxing 200 yards before climbing up through the trees. In a couple of places, minor unmarked trails drop to your left—continue on the main trail, heading generally northeast.

Almost 3 miles into the hike, the route turns east, then southeast as it contours up through the trees. You'll come to a sharp hairpin bend with a side trail heading due south (your right), barred from the main trail by a row of stones. If you take this fairly flat side trail due south for about 0.2 mile, you'll reach a saddle at about 5,600 feet elevation, with stunning views of Tucson. In fact, for many hikers this is a destination in itself, and they'll retrace their steps to the trailhead for an out-and-back hike of about 6 miles.

Back at the hairpin bend, you find yourself swinging north and then northeast, and as you climb you'll start noticing some strange assemblies of plants—I saw ferns growing around prickly pears and yuccas, shadowed by pine and oak trees with mistletoe growing on them. The trail continues to be quite clear, but there are some sections of loose rocks here. Vistas of cliffs and spires dominate the view to the north, while Tucson can be seen to the south.

About 4.5 miles into your hike, you'll reach the first trail sign since you began—you're almost at your goal! The sign indicates Finger Rock Trail #42 going right (east) for another 2 miles to its intersection with the Ventana Trail, and Pima Canyon Trail #62 going left (north). If you're really pooped, you could take Finger Rock Trail for about 50 yards to a drop-off with good views of Romero Canyon and Mount Lemmon. To reach Mount Kimball, however, you need to take the Pima Canyon Trail, which is actually a little less steep than the hike has been thus far. The trail sign is at 6,850 feet elevation, so you have only another 400 feet to gain.

As you set out on the Pima Canyon Trail, you'll immediately see views of the rounded peak of Mount Kimball to the northwest. After about 0.5 mile, the trail reaches a saddle with two small rock cairns on either side of the path (pranksters occasionally remove one). Here, turn right (north) onto a short trail that follows the pine-forested crest of Mount Kimball to a viewpoint—don't stop here, because there's a better view to come. Continue right for another 100 yards or so until you come to a dining table–sized boulder that marks the summit. Immediately behind it is a lovely rocky outcrop upon which you can rest and take in the expansive views, which stretch from the southwest to north and around to the southeast.

Major landmarks include Picacho Peak, sitting alone in the desert at 290° northwest; the white domes of the Biosphere, almost due north; Mount Lemmon, to the northeast; and, to the southeast, Tanque Verde Ridge and Mica Mountain, which at 8,666 feet is the highest peak in the Rincons. Don't forget to look straight down over the northern edge of the rocky outcrop to catch sight of an elegantly thin rock spire rising 100 feet up out of the forest.

Mount Kimball was named after Frederick Kimball, an Arizona state senator who helped develop Summerhaven as a summer getaway for Tucsonans during the first three decades of the 20th century. He was also a supporter of preservation and conservation in the Catalinas.

Most hikers return the way they came, though alternatively you can continue on the Pima Canyon Trail to the Pima Canyon Trailhead, 7.1 miles away, for a tough 12.2-mile trip that requires a car shuttle.

Nearby Attractions

See Hike 22, Pontatoc Ridge Trail (page 164).

Directions

See directions for Hike 22—the same parking area is used.

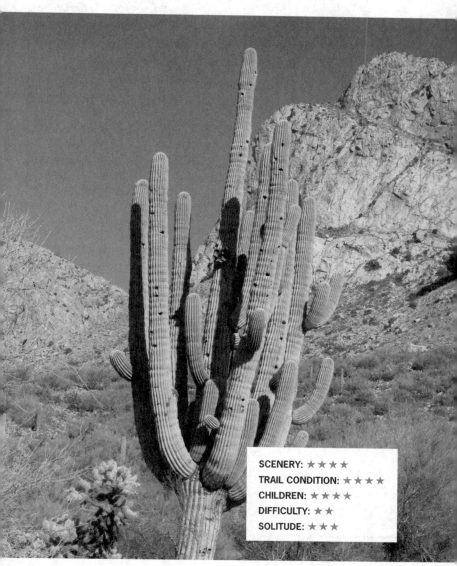

SCENERY: ★ ★ ★ ★
TRAIL CONDITION: ★ ★ ★ ★
CHILDREN: ★ ★ ★ ★
DIFFICULTY: ★ ★
SOLITUDE: ★ ★ ★

MANY-ARMED SAGUARO WITH PUSCH PEAK IN THE DISTANCE

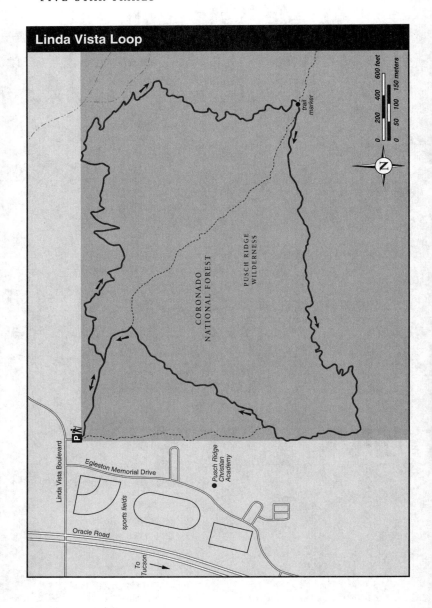

Linda Vista Loop

CORONADO NATIONAL FOREST

PUSCH RIDGE WILDERNESS

trail marker

0   200   400   600 feet
0   50   100   150 meters

N

Linda Vista Boulevard

Egleston Memorial Drive

sports fields

Pusch Ridge Christian Academy

Oracle Road

To Tucson

GPS TRAILHEAD COORDINATES: N32° 22.834' W110° 57.665'

DISTANCE AND CONFIGURATION: 3-mile loop

HIKING TIME: 1.5 hours

HIGHLIGHTS: Palo verde and cactus forest, views of Pusch Peak

ELEVATION: 2,675' at trailhead, 3,070' at high point

ACCESS: Parking area open 5 a.m.–9 p.m.; overnight parking permit available from Oro Valley Parks and Recreation, 520-229-5050; free

MAPS: Green Trails *Map 2886S–Santa Catalina Mountains*

FACILITIES: Parking for about 10 cars

WHEELCHAIR ACCESS: None

COMMENTS: No dogs or bikes allowed; horses permitted but infrequently seen

CONTACTS: Coronado National Forest, 520-749-8700, **www.fs.usda.gov/coronado**

Overview

Linda Vista (Spanish for "lovely view") is a fun, easy loop with attractive views of Pusch Peak at the western end of the Santa Catalina mountain range. The desert vegetation is thick, beautiful, and varied. Folks living in Tucson's northwest sector will find this an easily reached backyard hike. Late afternoon provides photographers with the best light for the mountains. The trail is narrow, and children need to be careful of prickly plants that grow up to the trail's edge.

Route Details

The trailhead has a map board and a choice of two routes going either east (left) or south (straight ahead). Both come back to this trailhead, and I describe the loop going east, making the longest possible hike. (Don't get confused by the map board at the trailhead, which has north pointing down instead of the more usual up.)

Immediately, superb views of Pusch Peak open in front of you, and you'll climb very gently for 0.14 mile to an unsigned Y-junction. Go left here—if you take the right fork, you'll cut almost a mile off the loop.

The trail approximately follows the boundary of Coronado National Forest, and you'll see some upscale houses to your left, one of which is covered with solar panels. (It never ceases to surprise me that so few houses in the Tucson area have solar panels—after all, this is one of the sunniest places in the USA.)

The trail traverses lush vegetation with many mature saguaro cacti, including one that has more than 25 arms—I lost count trying to get an accurate number. Keep your eyes open for it about 0.3 mile along the trail. You'll also see several kinds of cholla cacti, prickly pears, ocotillos, and many palo verde trees.

Palo verde is Spanish for "green stick," and these trees are unusual in having a green bark that can photosynthesize. Most trees have green leaves for photosynthesis, but palo verdes, found only in the desert Southwest, bear the tiniest of leaflets and rely on their green bark to compensate. It's a wonderful example of a tree adapting to its arid environment. In 1954, Arizona proclaimed the palo verde as its state tree.

During April and into May at higher elevations, palo verdes have a colorful blooming season, with thousands of small yellow flowers changing the bare green branches into lovely golden boughs. If you look carefully enough, you might see a small yellow crab spider camouflaged to look like a flower; these spiders don't make webs but instead lie in wait for insects feeding on nectar. Once the bloom is over, pollinated flowers develop into dangling seedpods that used to be an important food source for the local Tohono O'Odham people, who ground the seeds in stone mortars to make flour.

Occasionally and briefly descending on its zigzagging eastward leg, the trail has one noticeable descent before it eventually turns right and heads south. On this southbound leg, a few false trails to your right (west) look as if they might head back to the trailhead, but they come to a viewpoint just a few yards away before petering out quickly. Meanwhile, the main trail meanders south and passes a rusty trail sign on the left. It's so rusted that nothing can be read on it, but you're now more than halfway around the loop.

Behind the rusty sign, a narrow trail climbs east to Pusch Peak—the Linda Vista Loop Trail continues west. (The trail to the mountain is not marked on any maps and is not described here.) Barely 0.1 mile beyond the rusty trail marker, the trail reaches an unsigned Y. Here, take the left fork to complete the loop. (The right fork goes straight back to the parking lot, in case you're in a hurry.)

The westward leg of the loop yields views of Oro Valley, a burgeoning suburban town. (With no offense to its 41,000 residents, you'll probably be casting a look over your shoulder for the prettier mountain views.) Descend toward a school as the trail heads north, almost reaching the boundaries of the school property. At a trail fork behind the school, you can go straight (north) for 0.3 mile to the trailhead, or you can take the right (northeast) fork to complete the longest loop through the cactus–palo verde forest. A few hundred yards farther is an unsigned T-junction. The right (east) trail goes up to the rusty trail sign. The left (west) trail leads to the parking lot, about 0.2 mile away.

Directions

Take Oracle Road (AZ 77), Tucson's major road going north from the west side of town, to Catalina State Park: From the intersection of Oracle and Grant Roads, drive north on Oracle to enter Oro Valley and reach Linda Vista Boulevard, 9.3 miles north of Grant Road. Turn right onto Linda Vista and drive 0.1 mile to the parking area and trailhead.

Pima Canyon Trail to Mount Kimball

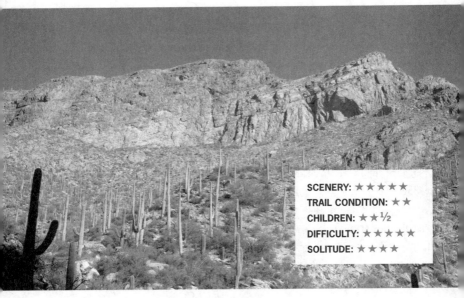

SCENERY: ★ ★ ★ ★ ★
TRAIL CONDITION: ★ ★
CHILDREN: ★ ★ ½
DIFFICULTY: ★ ★ ★ ★ ★
SOLITUDE: ★ ★ ★ ★

VIEW OF PUSCH PEAK FROM LOWER PIMA CANYON

GPS TRAILHEAD COORDINATES: N32° 31.205' W110° 56.871'

DISTANCE AND CONFIGURATION: 14-mile out-and-back

HIKING TIME: 10 hours

HIGHLIGHTS: Superb views; 2 small dams attracting wildlife; summiting a peak

ELEVATION: 2,920' at trailhead, 7,258' at Mount Kimball

ACCESS: Trailhead parking open 5 a.m.–9 p.m. daily, 24/7 pedestrian access; free

MAPS: Green Trails *Map 2886S–Santa Catalina Mountains*, USFS *Pusch Ridge Wilderness*, USGS *Tucson North*

FACILITIES: Parking for about 35 vehicles (may fill up on spring weekends); water fountain at trailhead; no restrooms

WHEELCHAIR ACCESS: Trailhead water fountain and signage only

COMMENTS: Horses permitted but rarely seen; dogs not allowed. Older maps predating late-20th-century housing developments show the trailhead farther east. Avid, fit hikers with two cars can climb up Finger Rock Trail and descend via Pima Canyon.

CONTACTS: Coronado National Forest, 520-749-8700, **www.fs.usda.gov/coronado**

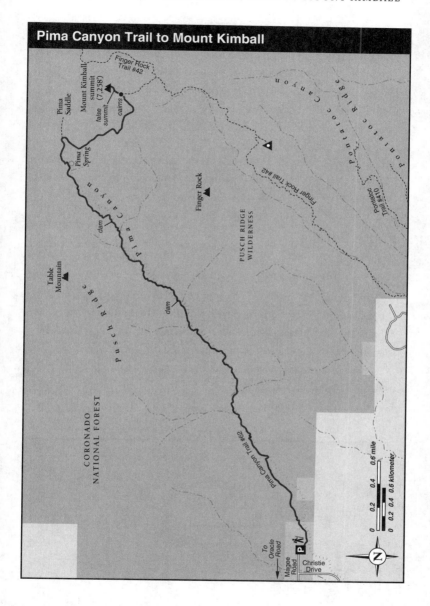

Pima Canyon Trail to Mount Kimball

Finger Rock Trail #42

Mount Kimball summit (7,258')

Pima Saddle

false summit

cairns

Pima Spring

Ponatoc Canyon

Ponatoc Ridge

Finger Rock

Finger Rock Trail #42

Pontatoc Trail #410

dam

Table Mountain

PUSCH RIDGE WILDERNESS

Pusch Ridge

dam

CORONADO NATIONAL FOREST

Pima Canyon Trail #62

To Oracle Road

Magee Road

Christie Drive

P

0   0.2   0.4   0.6 mile

0   0.2   0.4   0.6 kilometer

N

Overview

This trail attracts many hikers on its lower part but fewer hikers in its difficult higher reaches than the more-iconic Finger Rock Trail or the ever-popular Sabino Canyon. Those who go high enjoy superb views, including the rarely seen back side of Finger Rock, before bagging the summit of Mount Kimball. Two small dams built to attract wildlife provide splashes of water, riparian plants, butterflies, and birds. I almost graded this hike a 2 for kids until I encountered a tough family group that included a 10-year-old boy, who told me it was "really, really hard, and we got lost, but Dad found the way."

Route Details

The attractive trailhead at the east end of the parking lot features monuments to former Pima County Supervisor Iris O. Dewhirst, after whom the trailhead is named and who helped maintain public access to Pima Canyon during housing development in the 1980s, and to Tom Bingham, who was also involved in preserving canyon access and who died in 1992 while rock-climbing alone in the canyon he loved.

The trail heads generally east, passing informative signs and scattered upscale homes, and soon dips under a bridge that carries Barrel Cactus Drive above hikers. Then it begins to climb steadily but not steeply, with views of most of Tucson to your right and saguaro forest to your left. Enter Pima Canyon fairly high on the left side as the trail swings northeast and away from the city.

After about a mile, the trail drops quite suddenly to cross the usually dry creek bed—this is about as far as many casual walkers go, and you'll see fewer people continuing on. To your left are photogenic views of the mountains of Pusch Ridge, which form the northern edge of Pima Canyon.

Hike along the right side of the creek bed for a few hundred yards, then cross again to the left side briefly before returning to the right side. This third crossing may have trickles of water (not in late spring and summer) and has a few short false trails. One of the middle trails continues to climb along the right side of the creek bed and above a lush area of mesquites.

Over the next mile you'll recross the creek, usually dry but sometimes flowing shallowly, another half-dozen times. Lovely riparian woodlands of mesquite and cottonwoods indicate that there is water underfoot, even if it is infrequently seen. As you climb higher, the canyon walls close in around you for a stretch before they open into a shallow basin.

About 2.5 miles from the trailhead, around 3,800 feet elevation, the woodlands give way to gorgeous high-desert vegetation dominated by stick-like ocotillos and staghorn chollas, spiky yuccas and agaves, and a variety of cacti. Soon the trail crosses some rocky slabs with cairns helping you find the way, and then it threads its way between two grapefruit-sized depressions in the rock. These are mortars, used centuries ago by Native American women to grind mesquite beans and other local plants.

A couple of hundred yards beyond the mortars, on a short side trail to the left, is a rock-and-mortar dam, some 5 feet high and 15 feet across, built about 50 years ago by Arizona Game and Fish to provide water for wildlife. Behind it there's almost always a small pool of water, which attracts butterflies, birds, amphibians, occasional deer, and who knows what else. This is a frequent turnaround spot for hikers looking for a shorter scenic trip; it's about 6 miles out-and-back.

Cairns indicate the main trail continuing northeast up Pima Canyon and gradually merging into oak woodlands. About a mile above the dam, the trail becomes thin, loose in places, and rather exposed. It's not very difficult, but a novice hiker with a fear of heights might want to turn back here, because it does get steeper and looser.

The trail drops suddenly and begins to cross the canyon for the umpteenth time, but this time it climbs a central buttress that splits the canyon before crossing the second arm. When you're all the way across, look for a second dam to your right—it blends into the rock and is easily missed. This one is a little bigger than the first, but it tends to get silted up more.

Above the second dam the clear trail climbs steeply, with great views looking back down the canyon. The trail becomes a little overgrown in places but can be clearly followed to Pima Spring, about a mile beyond the dam. There's a small concrete holding tank below you to the left of the trail and, about 20 yards farther, another tank above you on the right.

LOOKING DOWN AT FINGER ROCK FROM ABOVE THE PIMA SADDLE TURNOFF

Above the spring, the trail gets steeper and looser. This is the most difficult section but is fairly clear, so most hikers have few problems as long as they concentrate on their footing. As you climb out of the canyon, you'll start to catch sight of Tucson again. Roughly half a steep mile beyond the spring, you'll reach a battered sign for Pima Saddle. If you have the energy, you can continue climbing straight on (east) for 0.25 mile to the saddle, or you can turn right on the trail to Mount Kimball, another 1.5 miles away.

The route, now contouring fairly flatly to the southwest, is fairly exposed. There are a couple of slightly washed-out spots where the trail is not immediately obvious, but you'll find it quickly enough a few yards on. Then swing around to the southeast, climbing up occasional cairned rocky slabs. Looking south (right), you'll get dramatic views of the back side of Finger Rock below you, with Tucson behind. Finally, the trail turns northeast, passes a false summit, and reaches the spectacular top. See Hike 19 (page 147) for descriptions of views from Mount Kimball.

Directions

From central Tucson, head north on Swan Road to Sunrise Drive and turn west (left) on Sunrise, which becomes Skyline Drive and then Ina Road. Almost 5 miles from Swan, you'll reach the intersection of Ina Road and First Avenue to the south and Christie Drive to the north. Turn right on Christie and follow it to Magee Road, where you turn right to reach the trailhead, 1.6 miles from Ina Road.

Alternatively, take Grant Road to First Avenue, drive north 6 miles to Ina Road, and cross Ina onto Christie Drive. Continue as described above.

From downtown, take Broadway east 1 mile to Euclid Avenue and turn left (north). After 2 miles, at Grant Road, Euclid Avenue becomes First Avenue; continue as described above.

From I-10, take Exit 248/Ina Road, drive east 6.3 miles to Christie Drive, and then turn left to reach the trailhead.

22 # Pontatoc Ridge Trail

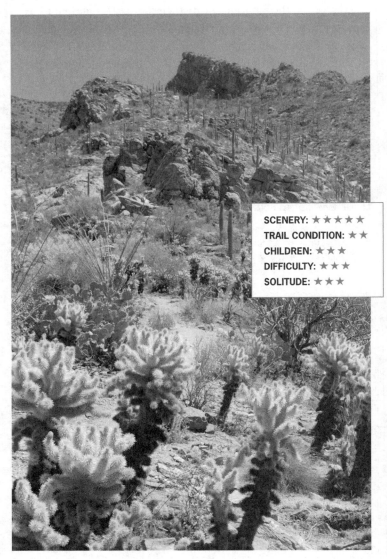

SCENERY: ★ ★ ★ ★ ★
TRAIL CONDITION: ★ ★
CHILDREN: ★ ★ ★
DIFFICULTY: ★ ★ ★
SOLITUDE: ★ ★ ★

TEDDY BEAR CHOLLAS ON THE PONTATOC RIDGE TRAIL

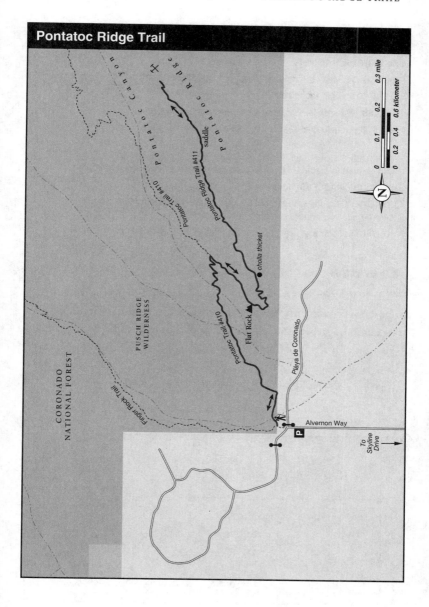

GPS TRAILHEAD COORDINATES: N32° 20.215' W110° 54.600'

DISTANCE AND CONFIGURATION: 5.2-mile out-and-back

HIKING TIME: 3.25 hours

HIGHLIGHTS: Views of Tucson and Finger Rock; teddy bear cholla thicket; old mine

ELEVATION: 3,100' at trailhead, 4,390' at trail's end

ACCESS: Trail open 24/7, parking lot open during daylight hours; no fee

MAPS: Green Trails *Map 2886S–Santa Catalina Mountains*, USFS *Pusch Ridge Wilderness*, USGS *Tucson North*

FACILITIES: Parking lot for 30 cars (no large vehicles) fills early on weekends; if it's full, overflow parking is available 0.2 mile back along Alvernon Way on gravel roadsides.

WHEELCHAIR ACCESS: None

COMMENTS: No dogs allowed. USFS trail signs and maps indicate that the trail is 2.6 miles one-way; my GPS reading was just under 2 miles.

CONTACTS: Coronado National Forest, 520-749-8700, **www.fs.usda.gov/coronado**

Overview

This trail affords excellent views of Tucson and its surrounding mountains from different angles—bring a city map and binoculars to pick out the streets and landmarks. Looking away from Tucson, you'll have superb vistas of Finger Rock (see Hike 19, page 147) and Pontatoc Canyon in the front ranges of the Santa Catalina Mountains. The hike ends at an old mine that gives the trail its name.

Route Details

The trailhead, at the north end of Alvernon Way, about 100 yards from the parking lot, is shared with the Finger Rock Trail (see page 147) and features informative notices about the bighorn mountain sheep that roam the area. Two very short, fairly steep switchbacks bring you to the signed trail fork where Finger Rock Trail #42 heads north and Pontatoc Trail #410 heads east (right).

Pick your way down a little drop-off where the trail isn't quite obvious: Look for it below you as it goes east, past a row of several upscale residences to the right of the trail. Within a few minutes the trail veers northeast, away from those nice-looking homes and into even-nicer-looking wilderness scenery, dominated by Finger Rock views to the north and Pontatoc Ridge, a roughly triangular, blocky-looking outcrop, to the east. Near the top of the ridge, you can see black caves that are the entrances to old mines.

About 0.6 mile from the trailhead, you'll cross a wash (dry almost always) and start climbing along the right side of the wash until you reach a signed fork 0.75 mile from the trailhead. Here, you could continue following the Pontatoc Trail—which goes straight (east) into Pontatoc Canyon for about 3 miles—or turn hard right (southwest) onto Pontatoc Ridge Trail #411, the hike described here.

The narrow trail flattens and looks down on the route you've just walked up. Almost 0.25 mile from the fork, you'll see large, flat, rocky areas to the right that are a perfect place to stretch out on for a snack while you admire the view of Tucson's west side. Downtown is about 8 miles away to the southwest, backed by the Tucson Mountains.

The trail continues southwest, past the flat rocks, for about 100 yards before it swings east and starts climbing, with ever-wider views of central Tucson. About 0.2 mile farther brings you to an unusually dense thicket of teddy bear cholla (*Opuntia bigelovii*), a cactus with a thick covering of golden spines. These will attach themselves to you with the merest touch, giving the plant the nickname "jumping cactus." Other closely related species are also known to jump . . . so beware!

Beyond the cholla thicket, the trail becomes indistinct in areas where it climbs rocky slabs. Watch for cairns to guide you, and ignore side trails that are crossed with a line of small rocks to indicate that they aren't the best way. Within a few minutes you should be on a distinct trail again, still climbing gently. To your left you'll see the Pontatoc Trail far below, wending its way up the canyon.

About 0.6 mile beyond the teddy bear chollas, the trail crosses a narrow saddle. Due south of the saddle, you'll have a great view of ruler-straight Swan Road traversing the east side of Tucson to Davis-Monthan Air Force Base, 10 miles away, and the Santa Rita Mountains beyond.

The narrow trail continues climbing Pontatoc Ridge for several hundred yards to a sign that oddly proclaims, "Dogs Prohibited Beyond This Point." (Dogs weren't allowed at the beginning of the trail, so I'm not sure how they got here to be prohibited again.) Above you, three cave-like openings to mine shafts are open but not maintained, and may be dangerous. The trail ends here, but you can scramble up short,

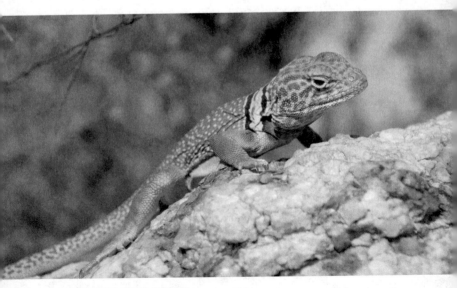

EASTERN COLLARED LIZARD

steep, loose paths to the mine openings and enter—a flashlight is useful. The mines, worked from 1906 to 1917, yielded small amounts of copper and silver.

Any exploration beyond the end of the trail is entirely at your own risk.

Nearby Attractions

The **DeGrazia Gallery in the Sun** (6300 N. Swan Rd.; 520-299-9191, **degrazia.org**) is 2 miles from the trailhead, near the intersection of Swan Road and Skyline Drive. This 10-acre National Historic District was the home and workplace of local artist Ted DeGrazia (1909–1982). The gallery grounds include a museum showcasing the painter's work, an adobe chapel, and other Southwestern architecture. A gift shop sells art books, posters, and knickknacks, and original pieces are available for purchase. Open daily, 10 a.m.–4 p.m., except January 1, Easter, Thanksgiving, and December 25; admission is free.

Directions

From central Tucson, head north on Swan Road to Skyline Drive, passing the DeGrazia Gallery to your right; turn left (west) on Skyline and drive 1 mile, then turn right (north) on Alvernon Way and drive 1 mile to the parking area. Alternatively, head north on Campbell Avenue to Skyline Drive, turn right (east), and drive 0.4 mile to where Skyline forks and becomes Sunrise Drive. Take the left fork to continue on Skyline another 0.7 mile to Alvernon Way, and turn left (north) to reach the parking area.

From I-10, take Exit 250/Orange Grove Road and drive 7 miles to Skyline Drive, then drive 1.1 miles to the fork with Sunrise Drive, continuing on Skyline to Alvernon.

Note: Alvernon Way, a main street crossing most of central Tucson, does not have a bridge across the Rillito River. Therefore, the trailhead must be approached from Skyline Drive, as described above.

23 Ventana Canyon to Maiden Pools and The Window

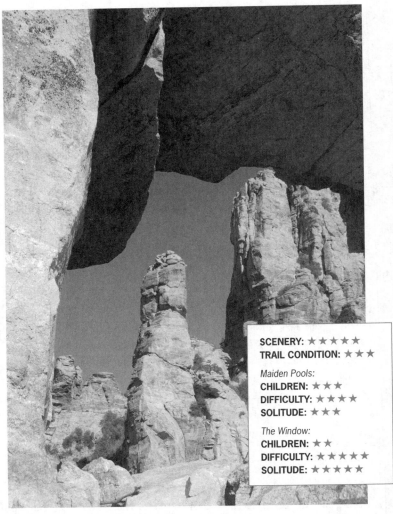

SCENERY: ★ ★ ★ ★ ★
TRAIL CONDITION: ★ ★ ★

Maiden Pools:
CHILDREN: ★ ★ ★
DIFFICULTY: ★ ★ ★ ★
SOLITUDE: ★ ★ ★

The Window:
CHILDREN: ★ ★
DIFFICULTY: ★ ★ ★ ★ ★
SOLITUDE: ★ ★ ★ ★ ★

THE SPIRES OF WINDOW PEAK, FRAMED BY THE WINDOW

Ventana Canyon to Maiden Pools and The Window

GPS TRAILHEAD COORDINATES: N32° 19.674' W110° 51.184'

DISTANCE AND CONFIGURATION: 4.6-mile out-and-back to Maiden Pools, 12.1-mile out-and-back to The Window

HIKING TIME: 3.5 hours to Maiden Pools, 10.5 hours to The Window

HIGHLIGHTS: Gorgeous canyon, pools, lush vegetation, birding, and an impressive geological formation

ELEVATION: 3,025' at trailhead, 4,300' at Maiden Pools, 7,000' at The Window

ACCESS: Trailhead open sunrise–sunset; free

MAPS: Green Trails *Map 2886S–Santa Catalina Mountains,* USFS *Pusch Ridge Wilderness,* USGS *Tucson North*

FACILITIES: Trailhead parking for about 25 cars; no large RVs

WHEELCHAIR ACCESS: None

COMMENTS: Hikers only. The Coronado National Forest trailhead map indicates 12.8 miles out-and-back to The Window, other maps show 13.2 miles, and previous guidebooks vary. My GPS showed 12.1 miles.

CONTACTS: Coronado National Forest, 520-749-8700, **www.fs.usda.gov/coronado**

Overview

The hike to Maiden Pools offers exceptional views of Ventana Canyon and is a fairly popular picnic destination. Above the pools, a less-traveled trail ascends through thriving woodlands to a ridge with views of Mount Lemmon and other landmarks. Keep going to a natural rock window, which makes for a satisfying destination and provides unusual photo ops.

Route Details

From the trailhead, you'll be forced to follow a narrow path for almost a mile, with chain-link fences on either side and forbidding No Trespassing signs. This is actually not as bad as it sounds: Thick vegetation and boisterous birdsong provide a good introduction to the trail, and hikers are happy that landowners were able to provide a corridor to the canyon. Even within this 15-foot-wide corridor, you'll cross a stream a few times as you ascend almost unnoticeably.

A switchback gateway, marking the border between private properties in Pima County and Coronado National Forest, is designed so that horses cannot pass. You come to a sign for Ventana Trail #98, beyond which the trail continues its gentle ascent, with a few more creek crossings. These are usually very straightforward, with rock slabs conveniently placed to keep your feet dry. In summer and late fall, the crossings are often dry, and they rarely fill to where you'll have to wade. In spring, you'll see butterflies along the creek.

Soon the canyon narrows, and dramatic rock cliffs and towers dominate the view. At times it feels as if you're surrounded by an Asian-mountain painting. About 1.5 miles into the hike, at around 3,400 feet elevation, you'll hit a series of switchbacks and find yourself climbing quite steeply. The trail is rocky but firm and clear, eventually topping out at a saddle at about 4,250 feet elevation.

Here, you're rewarded with a great view to the south of the eastern reaches of growing Tucson. The flat area in the middle distance is the Davis-Monthan Air Force Base, with Mount Wrightson and the Santa Ritas dominating the horizon. A couple of flat places on the saddle are good spots for a picnic. Beyond, the trail drops a few hundred yards to the Maiden Pools.

The pools are on the right side of the trail and extend for several hundred yards. Some are linked by pretty little waterfalls, and social side trails give access to a few (but not all) of the pools. After extended dry periods, such as June–July, before the monsoons, and November–December, before the winter snowmelt, the pools are mainly dry.

Above the pools, the thick vegetation attests that there's water in the canyon for most of the year. Oak trees are common, with occasional aspens, sycamores, and cottonwoods livening up the mix and many smaller bushes grabbing at your legs. The trail ascends in fits and starts, with a switchback here and a step-up there, interspersed with unexpected flat areas or descents to the creek, which is crossed several times. The underbrush occasionally makes the trail a little unclear, but helpfully placed cairns will guide you.

Eventually, there are more steep sections than flat ones, and you encounter loose trail underfoot. If you pay attention to your surroundings, you'll see a jagged cliff on the northeastern horizon, and for a few hundred yards you can make out the natural rock window that gives the canyon its name—*ventana* is Spanish for "window." From this angle, ascending to The Window looks like an epic rock climb, but you'll not need ropes, as hikers approach the window from the far side. Later on the trail, the view of The Window is hidden.

As you climb higher, pine trees begin to introduce themselves in the oak woodland. To your left, just south of west, you can appreciate the cliffs of the north face of Mount Kimball (see pages 147 and 158). You reach a trail junction at about 5 miles from the trailhead, with a metal marker indicating the Finger Rock Trail going left (west) and the Esperero Trail going right (northeast).

This is actually the end of the Ventana Trail—continue on the Esperero Trail for about another mile. It's steep enough that rock steps have been built into it at several points, and at one point the trail heads west for about 0.1 mile, which might make you think you're heading the wrong way. Fear not: It switches back and reaches a wonderful, almost flat ridge that you follow to the east, with views of Tucson to your right and Mount Lemmon to your left. This in itself is a great end to a hike, but the best is yet to come.

The final push is a few hundred yards of climbing, generally southeast, toward and then behind the rock buttress that houses The Window. You can't see this natural rock arch until you've almost passed it, so as you ascend the steep, loose trail behind the buttress, make sure to keep looking to your right.

The Window itself is about 15 feet high and 25 feet wide. Every time I go up there it's really windy, so hold on to your hat. Views to the west include Mount Kimball, Ventana Canyon, and much of Tucson; as you look the other way, the spires of Window Peak dominate the view. Just remember that the west side of The Window is a vertical cliff—so explore with care.

Directions

From I-10, take Exit 248/Ina Road and head east. After 6.8 miles, Ina becomes Skyline Drive and, almost 2 miles farther, becomes Sunrise Drive. Follow Sunrise about 6 miles to Kolb Road and turn left (north). Follow Kolb Road about 1.25 miles, passing the entrance to Loews Ventana Canyon Resort on your right and then taking the next right onto Resort Drive. Drive 0.1 mile to the employee parking lot on your left, and then drive through this lot to the fenced-off area designated for trailhead parking.

From most parts of Tucson, drive east to Kolb Road and turn left (north) on Kolb to its intersection with Tanque Verde Road. Turn right (east) on Tanque Verde, drive 0.6 mile, and then turn left (north) on Sabino Canyon Road. After 2.25 miles, Sabino Canyon becomes Kolb Road, which you follow north for just over 2 miles to Sunrise Drive. Keep going north on Kolb another 1.25 miles, and continue as described above.

Saguaro National Park West and Tucson Mountains (Hikes 24–29)

Saguaro
National Park West
and Tucson Mountains

FLOWERING SAGUARO

24 Saguaro National Park West:

Hugh Norris Trail to Wasson Peak

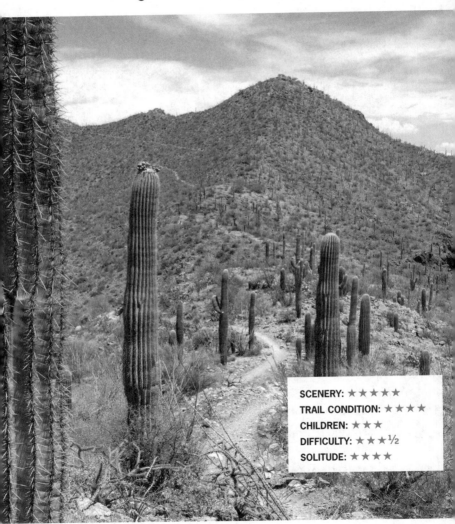

SCENERY: ★ ★ ★ ★ ★
TRAIL CONDITION: ★ ★ ★ ★
CHILDREN: ★ ★ ★
DIFFICULTY: ★ ★ ★ ½
SOLITUDE: ★ ★ ★ ★

SAGUAROS FOLLOW THE TRAIL TO THE RIDGE.

Saguaro National Park West: Hugh Norris Trail to Wasson Peak

GPS TRAILHEAD COORDINATES: N32° 16.286' W111° 12.182'

DISTANCE AND CONFIGURATION: 9.8-mile out-and-back

HIKING TIME: 5 hours

HIGHLIGHTS: Ridge views, desert flora, great 360° vistas from Wasson Peak

ELEVATION: 2,575' at trailhead, 4,687' at Wasson Peak

ACCESS: Trailhead open sunrise–sunset. Admission: $10/$5 per car/pedestrian, payable at the visitor center (2.5 miles away), valid for 1 week in both Saguaro National Park (SNP) districts; $25 for 1-year car pass. All National Park Service annual passes accepted.

MAPS: National Geographic–Trails Illustrated *237–Saguaro National Park,* Green Trails *Map 2910S–Saguaro;* free trail map available at visitor center

FACILITIES: Parking for 8 vehicles (no RVs or trailers) at trailhead and across the road; visitor center. See Nearby Attractions for an alternate trailhead.

WHEELCHAIR ACCESS: None

COMMENTS: The unpaved access loop closes at sunset, so don't get caught! This is a hikers-only trail.

CONTACTS: SNP Red Hills Visitor Center, 520-733-5158/5100, **nps.gov/sagu**

Overview

This is the longest trail in the Tucson Mountain (West) District of Saguaro National Park. Much of the beginning of the route involves hiking up shallow steps, but once you reach the long ridge, superb views unfold in all directions. The trail is clear, and it's almost impossible to get lost. Wasson Peak is the highest peak in the Tucson Mountains.

Route Details

The trail, named after a Tohono O'odham police chief who worked in the San Xavier Reservation in the 1930s, goes east from the tiny parking lot and, with minor exceptions, continues roughly east the whole way. If you leave in the morning to avoid the afternoon heat, you'll be facing the sun—don't forget your sunglasses!

Climbing up long but shallow steps with stone risers, you'll pass a trail register on your left after 100 yards where you're encouraged to sign in. Almost immediately, if the sky is clear, there are views of the white domes of the Kitt Peak observatories on the horizon about 32 miles to the southwest and, farther south, the distinctive triangular Baboquivari Peak, a sacred mountain for the Tohono O'odham people.

About 0.3 mile from the trailhead, the trail drops briefly south, crosses a sandy wash, and then continues east, still climbing the easy, loping steps up a valley. You're surrounded by as thick a stand of saguaros as you'll see anywhere. The trail climbs gradually, with occasional switchbacks, to a saddle at about 3,150 feet and 0.6 mile from the sandy wash. If you've been counting, you'll have climbed more than 700 steps from the trailhead to the saddle, and there will be far fewer steps ahead.

From this first saddle, you catch sight of the trail curving around fairly flatly to the right and several hundred yards in front of you. Behind you, to the west, you can see the farmlands of the Avra Valley. The rectangular water ponds in the valley are a groundwater-recharging facility run by Tucson Water, using CAP (Central Arizona Project) water channeled from the Colorado River via canals and pipelines. The trail swings briefly south as it continues with more steps through a garden-like area of truck-sized granite boulders scattered around, inviting exploration.

Soon you're heading back east, finally walking along a trail without steps—this is the trail you could see from the first saddle. To your north, beyond the well-defined boundary of the protected area of the national park, are views of the houses and trailers of the Picture Rocks area of the Avra Valley, along with various mountains rising out of the flat desert floor. Two conical formations near a mining area are named Twin Peaks; to their right lies the double-ended mountain of Panther Peak and Safford Peak, and to the far distant northwest is the steep profile of Picacho Peak.

The trail rises almost imperceptibly for a while and then makes a few quick switchbacks to arrive at a second saddle, at about 3,350 feet elevation and 0.7 mile from the first saddle. Suddenly, you get a view over the ridge to the south—the building with the curved front and parking lot, just over a mile away and 800 feet below you, is Saguaro National Park's Red Hills Visitor Center.

Now, the rocky but clear and well-graded trail tends to stay on or near the top of the ridge, with changing views to south and north. After climbing for roughly 0.7 mile, the trail descends and, as you go down, you'll see the grounds of the Arizona-Sonora Desert Museum

OCOTILLOS, PANTHER PEAK (LEFT), AND SAFFORD PEAK

in the valley to the southeast and, behind it on the horizon, Mount Wrightson, the highest peak in southern Arizona. Just past the point where the trail starts to climb again, a fenced-in abandoned mine is seen on the right. As with the many other old mines in the Tucson Mountains, entering is dangerous and strongly discouraged.

The trail continues about 0.2 mile beyond the mine to a well-signed intersection with the Esperanza Trail. Beyond, the trail climbs steadily but easily, with rocky and sandy footing, some flattish stretches, occasional dips, and sporadic steps. Much of the area is accented by the red flowers of ocotillo, mixed in with agaves and cholla cacti, during April and May.

The mountain ahead of you looks steep but is easily climbed, with 10 well-graded switchbacks leading to a high saddle that throws open views of all of Tucson below you. The distance from the Esperanza Trail intersection to this saddle is almost 2 miles. Barely 25 yards beyond is a marker for the King Canyon Trail, where you turn left and continue an easy 0.3 mile to the summit, with views of the Tucson basin to the east, surrounded by the Catalina, Rincon, and Santa Rita mountain ranges. (The King Canyon Trail heads right and descends to the pass, where it joins the Sweetwater Trail, covered in the next hike.) There is a trail register 100 yards before the summit of Wasson Peak.

The peak was named after John A. Wasson, a co-founder and controversial early editor of the *Arizona Citizen* newspaper, which later became the *Tucson Citizen* and now is an online magazine.

Nearby Attractions

The **Arizona-Sonora Desert Museum** (2021 N. Kinney Rd.) is justifiably the best "museum" in southern Arizona. Most of it is outdoors, with exhibits showing off the plants and animals of the Arizona-Sonora desert. There's much to see here: Two walk-in aviaries bring you close to hummingbirds and orioles; winding trails separate you from javelinas with almost invisible electronic fences; caves have secret passages that kids can squirm through; aquariums and terrariums surprise you with desert creatures. The museum has snack bars and an upscale restaurant as well. Admission: $19.50 adults, $6 ages 4–12; more information: 520-883-2702, **desertmuseum.org.**

The **Esperanza Trailhead** is 2.75 miles north and then east of the Hugh Norris Trailhead. The parking area here accommodates horse trailers and about 20 cars and has an accessible restroom; the Ez-Kim-In-Zin Picnic Area is across the road. The Esperanza Trail climbs 1.7 miles to the intersection with the Hugh Norris Trail, then drops 1.4 miles to the Mam-A-Gah Picnic Area on the Kings Canyon Trail. If you've had the bad luck of not getting a parking spot at the Hugh Norris Trailhead, you'll almost certainly get one here, and you can hike to Wasson Peak on this shorter, steeper trail.

Directions

Drive west on Speedway Boulevard, one of Tucson's longest and most important east–west thoroughfares. (I-10 intersects Speedway at Exit 257.) Speedway becomes Gates Pass Road at Camino de Oeste, 4.8 miles west of I-10. Continue 4.6 miles on Gates Pass Road, over Gates Pass (no trailers or RVs allowed), to its intersection with Kinney Road. Turn right on Kinney, passing the Arizona-Sonora Desert Museum, to reach the Red Hills Visitor Center after almost 5 miles. From the visitor center, it's another 1.6 miles to Hohokam Road, where you turn right onto an unpaved loop road and drive 0.8 mile to the trailhead. *Note:* Beyond the trailhead, Hohokam Road is one-way northeast for a couple of miles, so don't try to arrive at the trailhead from the north.

25

Saguaro National Park West:
Sweetwater Trail to Wasson Peak

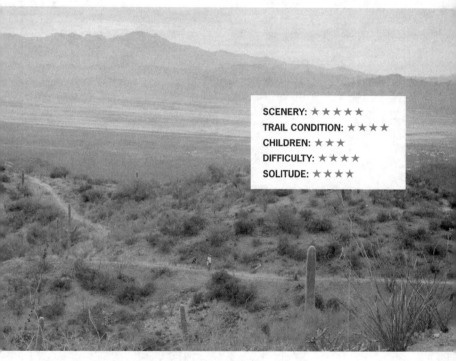

SCENERY: ★ ★ ★ ★ ★
TRAIL CONDITION: ★ ★ ★ ★
CHILDREN: ★ ★
DIFFICULTY: ★ ★ ★ ★
SOLITUDE: ★ ★ ★ ★

VIEW FROM THE PASS TOWARD KING CANYON TRAIL

GPS TRAILHEAD COORDINATES: N32° 17.326' W111° 07.259'

DISTANCE AND CONFIGURATION: 6.4-mile out-and-back to pass at end of Sweetwater Trail, 8.8-mile out-and-back to Wasson Peak

HIKING TIME: 3.25 hours to pass, 4.5 hours to Wasson Peak

HIGHLIGHTS: Classic Sonoran Desert flora and scenery in the lower part; views of Tucson in the distance; nice vistas from the pass and fabulous 360° views from Wasson Peak

ELEVATION: 2,810' at trailhead, 3,870' at pass, 4,687' at Wasson Peak

ACCESS: Trail open 24/7; park open sunrise–sunset. This is formally part of Saguaro National Park West, for which admission is $10/$5 per car/pedestrian, valid for 1 week

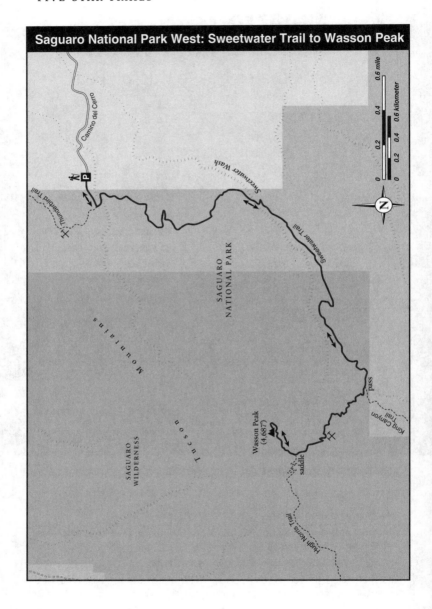

Saguaro National Park West: Sweetwater Trail to Wasson Peak

in both Saguaro National Park (SNP) districts; $25 for 1-year car pass; all National Park Service annual passes accepted. Note, however, that there is nowhere to pay nearby—the visitor center (2700 N. Kinney Rd.) is an hour's drive away.

MAPS: National Geographic–Trails Illustrated *237–Saguaro National Park*, Green Trails *Map 2910S–Saguaro*; free trail map available at visitor center

FACILITIES: None except for parking (about 20 cars and a couple of horse trailers)

WHEELCHAIR ACCESS: None

COMMENTS: Horses are permitted as far as the pass, but rarely encountered; no dogs, pets, camping, or mountain bikes allowed. This route is waterless and extremely hot in summer.

CONTACTS: SNP Red Hills Visitor Center, 520-733-5158/5100, **nps.gov/sagu**

Overview

Of the four main routes to Wasson Peak, the Sweetwater Trail is the least crowded and the second longest. The hike is relatively gentle to the pass, which marks the end of the Sweetwater Trail and where there are fine views to north and south. It's a satisfying destination for hikers with younger children or those with limited time. If you can continue on the steeper section to Wasson Peak, the panorama is definitely rewarding.

Route Details

At the west end of the parking area, the trailhead has a sign for trails to Wasson Peak. Walk west on a flat, rocky trail, soon passing a Saguaro National Park sign and map indicating the park boundary. At a trail register and signed T-junction 0.2 mile from the parking area, turn left (south) onto the wide and obvious Sweetwater Trail.

The trail soon swings southeast and crosses a dry wash, with plenty of loose rocks and pebbles, and generally continues climbing slightly to the south, with a couple of minor descents crossing washes taking you southwest or southeast. Occasionally, stairs are built into the trail as much as to control erosion as to help the hiker. The desert vegetation is thick with saguaros and other cacti, intermingled with a cornucopia of low trees and bushes. After an appropriately moist winter, you can expect spring wildflowers, though if the winter has been dry there won't be much of a bloom.

A little over a mile from the trailhead, you'll catch distant but notable views of Tucson, including downtown, to your left (east). These views last for a short while as the trail flattens and then begins a gentle descent, at times paralleling the wire fence of the national-park boundary.

You'll cross a small but steep little wash, which may have water flowing in it briefly after a monsoon rain. Stone stairs guide you up the southern side of the wash, which I'm guessing is the "Sweetwater" that the trail is named after—it's the largest watercourse on the trail. (About 2 miles east of here, Pima County recently protected more than 700 acres as the Sweetwater Preserve, where mountain biking and hiking trails can be accessed from the southern end of Tortolita Road.)

Now the trail climbs steadily southwest, with the "Sweetwater" valley below and to the right. Views open toward the north, with Wasson Peak on the western horizon. The Sweetwater Trail ends at the 3,870-foot-high pass, where it enters the King Canyon Trail. From the pass, the King Canyon Trail (see Nearby Attractions) winds off down to the southwest, with the grounds of the Arizona-Sonora

Desert Museum visible more than 2 miles away and more than 1,000 feet lower in the valley.

The pass provides good views but isn't much of a picnic spot if you're planning to stop here and return. There are no convenient rocks to sit on, and you'll have to picnic sitting on the dirt or standing up.

If you're ready to continue to Wasson Peak, 1.2 steeper miles farther, continue west and then northwest along the King Canyon Trail, which climbs narrowly and rockily from the pass. A sign indicates that this is a "Foot Trail Only—No Stock." As the inclination increases, the trail starts switchbacking and passes a closed-off mine shaft about 0.7 mile above the pass. In another 0.2 mile, the King Canyon Trail intersects the Hugh Norris Trail and turns right (northeast).

The final 0.3 mile is an easy ridge walk along the ending section of the Hugh Norris Trail (see previous hike) to the summit of Wasson Peak (4,687 feet). This is the highest point in the Tucson Mountains, and while it's low compared with the other ranges surrounding the city, it affords exceptional views looking up and around the horizon. A map and compass will help you identify some of the more prominent peaks.

Nearby Attractions

The **King Canyon Trail** also reaches the 3,870-foot-high pass described above. The trailhead for the King Canyon Trail is on the right (north) side of Kinney Road, 100 yards past the entrance to the Arizona-Sonora Desert Museum coming from Tucson. There is a dirt parking area for about 15 cars, but no other facilities. Follow signs for the Mam-A-Gah Picnic Area, which is accessible along a rocky road for hikers and equestrians only, 0.9 mile from the trailhead. Mam-A-Gah, with a pit toilet and a half-dozen picnic tables, is passed to your left; it's another 1.4 miles on a good, clear, rocky trail to the pass. At 7 miles out-and-back, this is the shortest route to Wasson Peak.

Directions

See next hike.

26

Saguaro National Park West:

Thunderbird Loop

> SCENERY: ★ ★ ★ ★
> TRAIL CONDITION: ★ ★ ★
> CHILDREN: ★ ★ ★
> DIFFICULTY: ★ ★ ★
> SOLITUDE: ★ ★ ★ ★

A SAGUARO ARM TOUCHES TWIN PEAKS AND POINTS TO PANTHER AND SAFFORD PEAKS.

GPS TRAILHEAD COORDINATES: N32° 17.326' W111° 07.259'

DISTANCE AND CONFIGURATION: 7-mile lollipop loop

HIKING TIME: 3.25 hours

HIGHLIGHTS: Thick Sonoran Desert flora and scenery at its best; old mines

ELEVATION: 2,810' at trailhead, 2,900' at high point, 2,450' at low point

ACCESS: This is formally part of Saguaro National Park West, for which admission is $10/$5 per car/pedestrian, valid for 1 week in both Saguaro National Park (SNP) districts; $25 for 1-year car pass; all National Park Service annual passes accepted. Note, however, that there is nowhere to pay nearby—the visitor center is an hour's drive away.

MAPS: National Geographic–Trails Illustrated *237–Saguaro National Park*, Green Trails *Map 2910S–Saguaro*; free trail map available at visitor center

FACILITIES: None except for parking (about 20 cars and a couple of horse trailers)

WHEELCHAIR ACCESS: None

COMMENTS: Horses are permitted but rarely encountered; no dogs, pets, camping, or mountain bikes allowed. Hiking distance is 7 miles on local maps, 6.2 miles according to my GPS.

CONTACTS: SNP Red Hills Visitor Center, 520-733-5158/5100, **nps.gov/sagu**

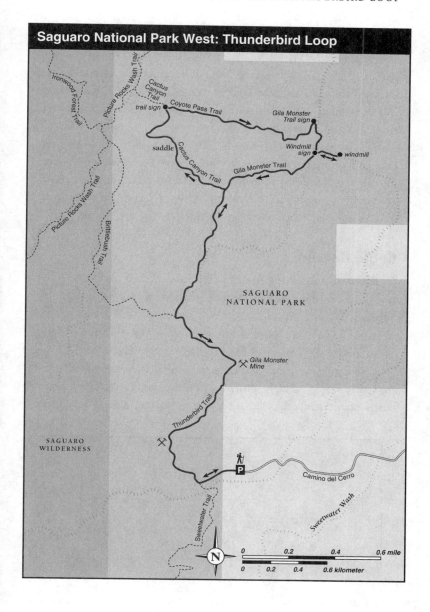

Saguaro National Park West: Thunderbird Loop

Overview

The Thunderbird Trail is the handle of this lollipop-shaped route, and at its end you'll do a loop along the attractively named Cactus Canyon, Coyote Pass, and Gila Monster Trails, which wind along valleys passing minor but scenic peaks. Along the way are several closed historic mines—it's illegal and dangerous to enter them, but it's thought-provoking to consider this part of the Southwest's heritage and wonder about what life must have been like for pioneering miners attempting to make a living without the conveniences of air-conditioning and cases of plastic bottles of water. Other sights to look for are cristate saguaros, spring flowers, and a windmill.

Route Details

At the west end of the parking area, the trailhead has a sign for trails to Wasson Peak. Walk west on a flat, rocky trail, soon passing a Saguaro National Park sign and a map indicating the park boundary. At a trail register and signed T-junction 0.2 mile from the parking area, turn right (northwest) onto the Thunderbird Trail.

The trail, rocky and wide enough for two, rises briefly, soon coming to its unexciting high point, and descends gently to a fork marked with a plain metal post. Perhaps it was once a trail sign. (A very short side trail rises to your left and comes to the first of many small mine shafts riddling the area.) The main trail continues north, then northeast, descending and very rocky, soon passing another mine on the left. You're now about 0.5 mile from the trailhead. Roughly 0.25 mile farther, you'll pass a rare cristate saguaro on your left—it's about 50 yards from the trail, so keep your eyes open to see it.

Still going gently downhill, you'll very briefly intersect the national-park boundary, marked with a wire fence and a sign telling you it's 0.9 mile back to El Camino del Cerro Road. A few hundred yards beyond, you'll reach the Gila Monster Mine, one of the biggest in the area and marked on some maps. Copper, lead, and zinc were the major minerals extracted here from two shafts roughly 10 yards apart. It's closed, as are all the mines in the area.

Several trails converge on this mine; you'll need to turn sharply left (northwest) just before the mine entrance and hike on a narrow, ascending trail. Soon the trail undulates up and down, one person wide, crossing minor washes, with saguaros of all sizes everywhere. About 0.5 mile from the Gila Monster Mine, the Brittlebush Trail diverges to the left (west) but is easy to miss. There is no sign, though there might be a pink plastic ribbon tied to a branch or a tiny pile of rocks marking the turn.

Our trail continues north and then north-northeast to a clear junction marked with a small pile of rocks. This is the unheralded end of the Thunderbird Trail, and if you look left (west) you'll see a sign less than a hundred yards away. It indicates the beginning of the Cactus Canyon Trail, your route to the Coyote Pass Trail 0.7 mile away.

The Cactus Canyon Trail soon crests a small saddle, and as it does you get lovely views of Panther and Safford Peaks (to the left and right) on the horizon about 3 miles to the northwest, with Picture Rocks Road in the valley below. Dropping from the saddle, you'll note more signs of mining activity and then reach a sign pointing out the beginning of Coyote Pass Trail, with Gila Monster Trail 0.8 mile away to the northeast and Picture Rocks Wash Trail 0.2 mile to the northwest. Turn right here.

The Coyote Pass Trail is fairly flat, following and occasionally crossing an almost-always-dry stream bed—to my mind, the least enjoyable part of the hike. Toward the end of this trail are several Trail Closed signs; stay on the sandy creek bed until the intersection with the signed Gila Monster Trail. This is the lowest part of the hike, and you'll be gently climbing most of the rest of the way.

Turn right (roughly south) on the Gila Monster Trail, following a dry wash about 15 feet wide. After 0.1 mile, a sign on the left of the wash says "Windmill." Tulips abound. A short side trail, maybe 300 yards or less, leads to a small, forgotten windmill perched over a concrete tank. One of the windmill blades reads "Aermotor USA." This Texas-based company has sold windmills since 1888 and continues to provide ranchers and homesteaders with windmills designed to pump groundwater.

Returning from the windmill side trip, you'll continue southwest along the wash bottom for 0.1 mile to a fork in the stream bed—here, take the right (west) fork. A bit over 100 yards along, the stream bed narrows and the left (south) bank becomes a 15-foot-high earthen cliff. Here, look for the trail leaving the stream bed on the right bank, heading northwest. There is no sign. Soon the Gila Monster Trail swings west, and you continue for about 0.3 mile, looking for the pile of rocks marking the north end of the Thunderbird Trail. (If you reach the sign for the Cactus Canyon Trail, you missed the Thunderbird Trail.) Turn left (south) on the Thunderbird Trail and retrace your footsteps along it to the parking area.

Nearby Attractions

The northern end of Saguaro National Park West has several more trails, such as the Brittlebush, Ringtail, Mule Deer, Picture Rocks Wash, and Ironwood Trails, which can be added to the loop I describe to make a longer day hike. Using a compass and one of the maps listed in the introduction to this hike will give you opportunities to explore further.

Directions

From downtown or midtown Tucson, drive west to I-10 and take the interstate north to Exit 252 for Ruthrauff Road and Camino del Cerro Road. From this exit, turn left (under the interstate) and drive west on Camino del Cerro Road for 5.6 miles to the parking area. The last 2.6 miles are twisty, but you'll see signs for either Camino del Cerro Road or Sweetwater Trail.

If you're driving from the Foothills north of Tucson, take Orange Grove Road west to La Cholla Boulevard. Turn left (south) and drive 2 miles to Ruthrauff Road, then turn right (west), drive 1 mile to I-10, and continue straight (west) on Camino del Cerro Road, as described above.

TYPICAL VEGETATION ON THE THUNDERBIRD LOOP

Sentinel Peak

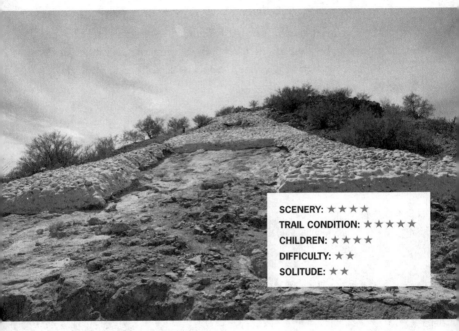

SCENERY: ★ ★ ★ ★
TRAIL CONDITION: ★ ★ ★ ★ ★
CHILDREN: ★ ★ ★ ★
DIFFICULTY: ★ ★
SOLITUDE: ★ ★

LOCALS CALL IT "A" MOUNTAIN.

GPS TRAILHEAD COORDINATES: N32° 12.826' W110° 59.9755'

DISTANCE AND CONFIGURATION: 4-mile lollipop from lower parking lot; much shorter from upper parking lot

HIKING TIME: 1.75 hours from lower parking lot

HIGHLIGHTS: Surrounding mountain vistas and great views of downtown Tucson

ELEVATION: 2,499' at lower parking lot, 2,766' at upper parking lot; 2,897' at Sentinel Peak

ACCESS: Daily, 9 a.m.–8 p.m., until 6 p.m. Sunday; free

MAPS: None besides the trail map provided here

FACILITIES: Two free parking lots, picnic bench; no restrooms

WHEELCHAIR ACCESS: 0.1 mile of trail from east end of upper parking lot to two signed overlooks

COMMENTS: Sentinel Peak is known locally as "A" Mountain. Leashed dogs permitted.

CONTACTS: Tucson Parks and Recreation, 520-791-5909, **tinyurl.com/tucsonparksandrec**

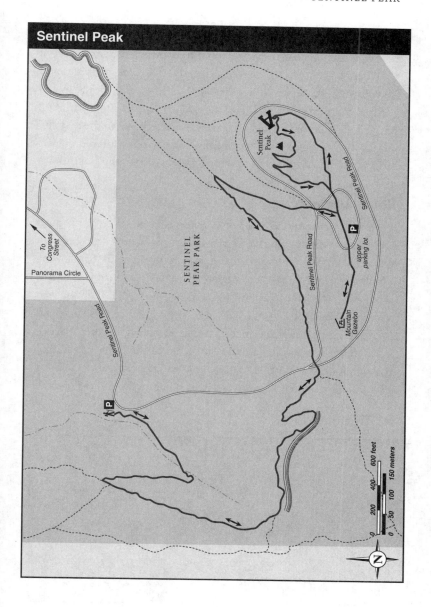

Sentinel Peak

Sentinel Peak

To Congress Street

Panorama Circle

Sentinel Peak Road

SENTINEL PEAK PARK

Sentinel Peak Road

Sentinel Peak Road

upper parking lot

Mountain Gazebo

0   200   400   600 feet

0   50   100   150 meters

N

Overview

Sentinel Peak, a small, outlying summit at the southeastern end of the Tucson Mountains, overlooks the city and gives great views of downtown and the whole city spreading out beyond, backed by the Santa Catalina and Rincon Mountains. Many visitors simply drive up to the upper parking lot and walk a few hundred yards to the best city views. My description starts from the lower parking lot and follows an easy, scenic trail through the upper parking lot to the summit.

Route Details

The huge letter *A* on the east side of Sentinel Peak, visible from much of Tucson, stands for the University of Arizona, whose students constructed and then whitewashed it on the mountain in 1915, following a football victory. Since then, students have whitewashed it annually, with a patriotic change to white, red, and blue after 9/11. It's even been colored green for St Patrick's Day! In recent years, Tucson's Parks and Recreation department has maintained and whitewashed the logo.

The trail leaves the southwest corner of the lower parking lot at a sign for the Gilbert Escandón Jiménez Trail, named in 2013 for a local resident and hiker who has been climbing the route for more than 70 years. The thin, rocky trail goes south and starts by parallel-ing the road to the upper parking lot. Look over your left shoulder for views of downtown. Very soon, the trail veers away from the road, and 0.1 mile later it hairpins, crossing a small gully.

As you climb the hairpins, the Santa Catalina Mountains come into view to the north. About 0.25 mile from the trailhead, you reach a T-junction where you turn left (south). An additional 0.3 mile takes you to a ridge from which you can see the southern end of the Tucson Mountains to the southwest and the Santa Ritas to the southeast. The trail follows this scenic ridge to the east and soon comes to a view of a hill topped with a stone gazebo, or ramada. This is the western end of Sentinel Peak, which is circumnavigated by a one-way road going past the A logo and the upper parking lot, though neither can be seen from this point.

The trail switchbacks down to the road, and you cross it at the point where the one-way loop around Sentinel Peak begins. Hiking along the road is not recommended because it is narrow and curving, and it has no pedestrian path. Instead, pick up the trail on the other side of the road and continue east on the left side of the lower part of the road. Very soon you'll pass a rustic memorial stone and cross for a man nicknamed Gibby who, presumably, loved the outdoors.

The trail is flat and rocky until about 0.3 mile from the road crossing, where it suddenly climbs steeply and briefly to the right and encounters a T-junction—here, turn right, roughly southwest and in the direction of the stone gazebo, climbing a rocky path to the road around Sentinel Peak. Cross the road and you'll see the entrance to the upper parking lot on your right.

From this parking lot you can head west a couple of hundred yards on a straight, flat path to the roofed stone gazebo, with wall benches, views, and a picnic bench and barbecue grill nearby. Alter-natively, find a signboard with a map of the area at the east end of the parking lot. From here, the 0.1-mile, wheelchair-accessible Mis-sion View Trail (completed in the fall of 2013) takes you to a couple of new lookout points with informative photo plaques describing

Tucson's history. Also from here, various signed trails lead the way to "A" Mountain, to the highest point of Sentinel Peak, and to a city overlook. None of these trails is more than 0.2 mile long, and despite the signs, it's easy to become confused by the decades of footprints that have been made by past visitors. Don't worry—you can't get lost.

Nearby Attractions

Downtown Tucson is experiencing a renaissance, with a new streetcar being completed as this book goes to press. The streetcar, which will link the University of Arizona with downtown via Fourth Avenue, should be running by early fall of 2014. **Fourth Avenue** prides itself on having numerous local eateries, drinking establishments, and eclectic shops without having one chain outfit. It completely closes to traffic twice a year for spring and winter street fairs (usually March and December), which seem to attract most of Tucson.

Congress Street also boasts a bunch of fine but offbeat restaurants, as well as music venues and the beautifully refurbished Fox Theatre, which looks the way it did when it opened in 1930. Streets nearby lead to the Tucson Convention Center, the Tucson Museum of Art and other museums, several theatres, and historic districts. The **Tucson Visitor Center** (110 S. Church St., Ste. 7199, in La Placita Village; 800-638-8350; **visittucson.org**) is a source of local information, as is this writer's own mobile app, **Tucson & the Old Southwest,** ($2.99), available at the iTunes Store and the Google Play Store.

Directions

From central Tucson, drive west on Broadway Boulevard to downtown, and where Broadway becomes one-way eastbound, cross downtown on Congress Street, one-way westbound. Continue on Congress Street under I-10 and, 0.8 mile beyond the freeway, turn left (south) on Cuesta Avenue. Drive up Cuesta for 0.6 mile to the lower parking lot, on your right. Here, Cuesta becomes Sentinel Peak Road, which goes to the upper parking lot.

If you're approaching downtown along I-10, take Exit 258 for Congress Street; drive west to Cuesta Avenue and continue as described in the previous paragraph.

VIEW OF DOWNTOWN TUCSON FROM SENTINEL PEAK

Tucson Mountain Park:
Brown Mountain Loop

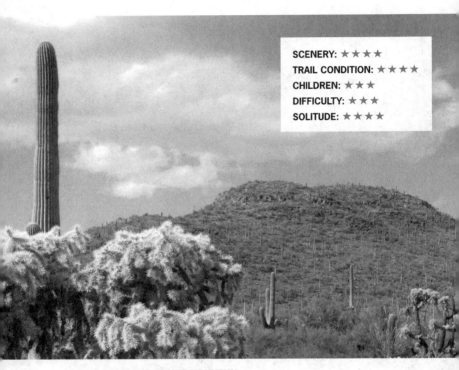

SCENERY: ★ ★ ★
TRAIL CONDITION: ★ ★ ★ ★
CHILDREN: ★ ★ ★
DIFFICULTY: ★ ★ ★
SOLITUDE: ★ ★ ★ ★

CHOLLA CACTI AND BROWN MOUNTAIN

GPS TRAILHEAD COORDINATES: N32° 13.778' W111° 08.706'

DISTANCE AND CONFIGURATION: 4.5-mile loop

HIKING TIME: 2.75 hours

HIGHLIGHTS: Ridge hike with views of desert and mountains

ELEVATION: 2,700' at trailhead, 3,098' at Brown Mountain

ACCESS: Open sunrise–sunset; free

MAPS: National Geographic–Trails Illustrated *237–Saguaro National Park*, Green Trails Map *2910S–Saguaro*

FACILITIES: The Brown Mountain Picnic Area has 4 picnic ramadas and grills; no water or restrooms. The Juan Santa Cruz Picnic Area has about a dozen picnic tables in varying states of repair, some shaded; restrooms and water fountain about 50 yards behind.

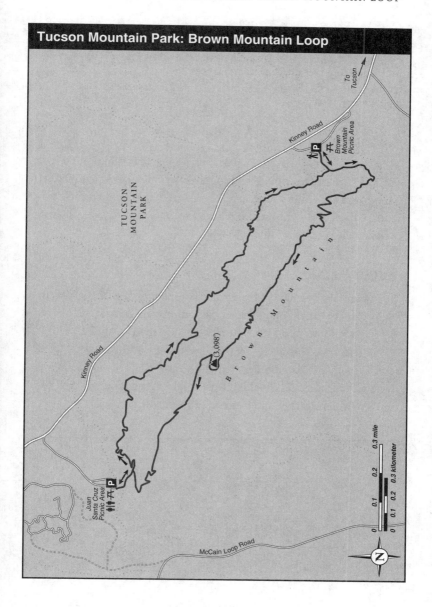

WHEELCHAIR ACCESS: Picnic areas only

COMMENTS: Horses are permitted but rarely seen; no dogs. This is a good hike from fall to spring, but it gets darned hot in the long Sonoran summer. Bring plenty of water—there is none available except at the Juan Santa Cruz Picnic Area.

CONTACTS: Pima County Natural Resources, Parks and Recreation, 520-877-6000, pima.gov/nrpr

Overview

It is satisfying to hike over and around an outlying mountain of the Tucson Mountains. You get to summit a minor peak, enjoy great views, and see plenty of desert plants, with a bonus of spring flowers in March and April. Trail signs are adequate, but occasionally you need to use your route-finding skills.

Route Details

The mountain was named for Cornelius Brown, first chairman of the Pima County Parks Commission. The commission was set up to oversee Tucson Mountain Park, which was established in April 1929.

I describe this hike clockwise, starting from the Brown Mountain Picnic Area, beginning with the gentle climb and traverse of Brown Mountain and finishing with a valley walk. You can pick the trail up from near the Juan Santa Cruz Picnic Area as well.

Brown Mountain Parking Area has four picnic ramadas spread over a few hundred yards; start from the third one if you've driven from Tucson. The trail leaves from behind a Tucson Mountain Park map sign, heading approximately west (bearing right, first northwest, then soon southwest). After 150 yards you'll cross a small wash (almost always dry), and a few yards later you'll reach an unsigned T-junction with a two-armed decapitated saguaro. This is the Brown Mountain Trail—turn left (south). After a few hundred yards, you'll see a sign reading "Cougar Trail 1.1," where you turn right and begin climbing roughly north. (If you cross the wash again, 20 yards beyond this sign, you missed the right turn.)

The trail climbs and switchbacks past saguaros in all stages of life, ranging from young ones less than a foot high to massive many-armed monarchs. Underfoot, multihued rocks are brownish-purple and salmon-colored. When you reach the summit ridge, you'll find an open area to the left of the trail where you can pause and take in the view to the southeast.

Old Tucson (see nearby attractions) lies to the east-southeast, with Gates Pass Road climbing above it. To the south-southeast is the Gilbert Ray Campground (the only one in Tucson Mountain Park, suitable mainly for RV campers), and gazing beyond it to the horizon you'll see the Santa Ritas and Mount Wrightson.

From here, the summit ridge climbs briefly north and then swings northwest, with super views on either side. Off in the distance to your left, about 40 miles to the southwest, you can see Kitt Peak with its telescopes; south of it is the distinctive triangular shape of Baboquivari Peak. On the other side of the ridge are the Tucson Mountains. The highest of several peaks along the ridge is marked as 3,098 feet on most maps, and from here you can see the Arizona-Sonora Desert Museum to the northwest.

After the highest peak, the trail drops and turns southeast for a short distance before hairpinning back to the northwest. The trail then climbs around the right (east) side of a final peak, without climbing it, then drops to a sign that appears seemingly in the middle of nowhere, directing you to the Gilbert Ray Campground, back the way you came, and the Juan Santa Cruz Picnic Area, which is your route.

About 200 yards beyond this sign, the trail reaches a T-junction. There is no sign here, but there is a flat rock slab about 2 feet square. Going right (east) continues along the base of the mountain to the Brown Mountain Picnic Area; going left (west) descends about 200 yards to the Juan Santa Cruz Picnic Area, which provides a restroom and a place to eat your snack or packed lunch. You've hiked almost 2.5 miles to this point. Some hikers prefer to retrace their steps from the northwest end of the mountain to enjoy the ridge views again.

Continuing east from the junction with the flat rock slab, follow the valley at the base of Brown Mountain. The trail meanders pleasantly, east and then generally southeast, with the mountain looming to the right. Desert flowers abound in spring, and vegetation is fairly thick year-round, so the trail never goes far in a straight line, instead twisting and turning around clumps of cactus or large rocks.

Almost 2 miles from the Juan Santa Cruz Picnic Area, a hard fork to the left (north) goes over a tiny, broken concrete dam—don't take this trail. Continue southeast, with your eyes open for the decapitated cactus you saw near the beginning of the hike. It's on the right side of the trail, about 100 yards beyond the fork over the dam. At the cactus, turn left (northeast) and return to the parking area, which is less than 200 yards away but not visible until you are almost back to your car.

Nearby Attractions

The movie studios at **Old Tucson** (201 S. Kinney Rd.; 520-883-0100, **oldtucson.com**) have been active for more than 70 years. John Wayne and many other actors shot their way to fame in Westerns made here. Today the studios are still used for filming but are also open as a tourist attraction, with actors performing stunts and mixing with the crowds. Gold panning, stagecoach rides, Wild West gun fights, and an old-time saloon are among the attractions. Admission: $16.95 for guests age 12 and over, $10.95 for kids ages 4–12, free for kids age 3 and younger; check the website for specific days and hours of operation.

See the next hike, Hike 24 (page 178), and Hike 25 (page 185) for other nearby attractions.

Directions

Drive west on Speedway Boulevard, one of Tucson's longest and most important east–west thoroughfares. (I-10 intersects Speedway at Exit 257.) Speedway becomes Gates Pass Road at Camino de Oeste, 4.8 miles west of I-10. Continue on Gates Pass Road for 4.6 miles, crossing Gates Pass (no RVs or trailers allowed). Where Gates Pass Road intersects Kinney Road, turn right on Kinney and drive 0.8 mile to the Brown Mountain Picnic Area, on your left.

If you have an RV or trailer, Kinney Road is reached on Ajo Way (AZ 86) from south Tucson. Ajo Way intersects I-10 at Exit 263 or I-19 at Exit 99; drive west from these exits and turn right from Ajo Way onto Kinney. From here it's about 6 miles to the Brown Mountain Picnic Area.

BARREL CACTI

Tucson Mountain Park:
Yetman Trail

| SCENERY: ★ ★ ★ ★ |
| TRAIL CONDITION: ★ ★ ★ |
| CHILDREN: ★ ★ ★ ★ |
| DIFFICULTY: ★ ★ ★ |
| SOLITUDE: ★ ★ ★ ★ |

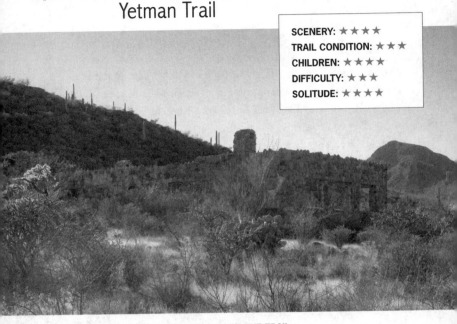

RUINS OF THE BOWEN HOUSE SEEN FROM THE TRAIL

GPS TRAILHEAD COORDINATES: N32° 13.045 W111° 06.176'

DISTANCE AND CONFIGURATION: 6-mile point-to-point with car shuttle, 12-mile out-and-back

HIKING TIME: 3 hours one-way

HIGHLIGHTS: Lowland Sonoran desert scenery with appealing cactus-covered mountains; following the steps of a TV personality

ELEVATION: 2,975' at western trailhead, 3,184' at high point, 2,662' at eastern trailhead

ACCESS: Open 24/7; free

MAPS: National Geographic–Trails Illustrated *237–Saguaro National Park,* Green Trails Map *2910S–Saguaro*

FACILITIES: None except for parking (about 10 or 14 cars at west or east end; no RVs or trailers)

WHEELCHAIR ACCESS: None

COMMENTS: This relatively flat desert trail is popular, but not crowded, with mountain bikers, many of whom know it well and are a good source of information. Horses are permitted but rarely seen. Dogs are prohibited, but that rule is frequently ignored. This is a good

Tucson Mountain Park: Yetman Trail

hike from fall to spring, but it gets darned hot in the long Sonoran summer. Bring plenty of water—there is none available anywhere.

CONTACTS: Pima County Natural Resources, Parks and Recreation, 520-877-6000, pima.gov/nrpr

Overview

There are no must-see views on this hike, which perhaps is what makes it attractive. The reliable views of thick stands of saguaros, prickly pear, cholla cacti (the "jumping" kind), ocotillo, palo verde, mesquite, and spring flowers, with a backdrop of numerous cliffs and crags at the south end of the Tucson Mountains, make this a wild-looking place. It's a hike that somehow grows on you.

Route Details

This route is described from the western Yetman Trailhead, slightly west of Gates Pass, hiking east to the Camino de Oeste Trailhead, which is 300 feet lower. Tucson Mountain Park trail signs tend to face the hiker leaving from the Yetman Trailhead, which makes it easier to navigate from this direction. The signs are not as high-quality as those found in state and federal areas and are subject to vandalism, so hikers should carry a map and compass if they don't know the trail well. There are numerous intersections with mapped and unmapped trails.

David Yetman worked to protect the environment as a member of the Pima County Board of Supervisors from 1977 to 1988, and this trail was named in his honor when he retired from politics. Since then he has worked with the Audubon Society and the University of Arizona, has authored numerous books, and has for several years served as the quirky host of the PBS television series *The Desert Speaks*, in which he explores the geology, wildlife, and inhabitants of American deserts from Arizona to Argentina.

Grab your water bottles and leave the southeastern corner of the parking lot on a wide, rocky trail that climbs gently southeast past a couple of trail signs. After 0.45 mile you'll conquer a pass— the high point of the trail, 3,184 feet on my GPS but marked variously on maps. Here, signs indicate the Golden Gate Trail to the right (returning to Gates Pass Road) and the Gates Pass Trail to the left (not shown on the maps I used).

The Yetman Trail forges on to the southeast, descending slowly. The peak to your right (west) is Golden Gate Mountain, 4,288 feet, the highest point in the southern half of the Tucson Mountains. Ahead (southeast) in the distance is the Tucson Estates housing development, beyond which the Santa Ritas lie on the horizon.

Thick stands of teddy bear cholla accompany the next section of trail. More than a mile from the trailhead, you'll angle left (east) at a sign for the Yetman Trail (going straight takes you to the Tucson Estates), and almost 1.5 miles from the trailhead another sign indicates that you fork east (west) again on the Yetman Trail. Just beyond here is an unsigned fork—here, bear left again.

The trail undulates and passes a sharp backward turn to the right, which you ignore; the route continues mainly east and is fairly flat. In this section of typical lowland desert scenery, a rare cristate saguaro cactus stands on the left. If you're one of those experienced (lucky?) hikers who can somehow both look around and keep your eyes on the rocky trail, you'll see it.

Almost 2 miles of rolling hiking, parts of it following a sandy wash that's almost always dry, bring you to the signed intersection with the Starr Pass Trail, where you bear left. Some maps indicate the Starr Pass Trail as the short Saguaro Rib Trail, which quickly brings you to the Starr Pass Trail. The trail is flat now and, about 200 yards later, reaches another sign for Starr Pass Trailhead 1.1, quickly followed by a sign for 36th Street Trailhead 0.9. (These trailheads provide access to equestrians.) The Yetman Trail bears left at both of these, heading east-southeast.

Soon the trail swings north and begins to climb gently, with super views of the southern end of the craggy Tucson Mountains to the left. About 0.6 mile from the previous signs, you reach a small pass with three trail junctions and a vandalized sign. Here, look for the thin, poorly marked Yetman Trail to the left (northwest). (Right, southeast,

WEATHERED SIGN AT THE YETMAN TRAILHEAD

follows the Rock Wren Trail to an equestrian trailhead. Straight on, northeast, is an unmapped trail that goes to a golf course.)

Climbing on the narrow Yetman Trail, you get glimpses of Tucson to the northeast. These views soon disappear as you hike up a quiet valley, then drop generally northwest, until about a mile from the previous turn, where you'll see a ruined stone house to the left. You can ignore the building and see it from the trail, or you can hike up and through it and meet up with the trail again a few hundred yards along.

If you hike through the house, the solid stone walls give you the impression that this was a good-sized place and would have been a comfortable home at one time. It was built in the 1930s by Sherry Bowen, an editor of the *Arizona Daily Star* who moved with his family to New York City in 1944. I don't know what happened after that, but the sturdy stone walls endured and are known today as the Bowen House.

Soon after the Bowen House, the trail swings northeast and follows a wide wash. In this area are several small signs that simply say "Trail." Look for an unmarked trail leaving from the right side of the sandy wash, which follows the right bank on a narrower but firmer footing. After a few hundred yards, this trail crosses the wash to the left bank, and four more crossings follow. Most of the year the wash is sandy and dry, so you could walk along it, but hiking along the banks is easier.

Eventually, the trail on the left side of the wash crosses an iron-pole gate indicating that you're leaving Tucson Mountain Park and entering private property. Buildings are visible. The trail soon crosses the wash one more time before arriving at the Camino de Oeste trailhead.

Nearby Attractions

Gates Pass (3,120 feet) was named after Thomas Gates, a Western pioneer whose well-rounded résumé included professional gambler, saloonkeeper, political lobbyist, historian, prison superintendent, and mine owner. His profitable carbonate mine, in the Waterman Mountains about 30 miles west of Tucson, led him to establish a route over a pass through the Tucson Mountains to shorten the journey from his claim to Tucson. The city was unable to come up with the funds to build a road, so in 1883 Gates funded it himself at a cost of $1,000.

The **Gates Pass Overlook** is a popular stop for drivers and hardy cyclists following the historic route. Heading west from Tucson, the overlook is on the right (north) side of the narrow, winding road (no commercial vehicles, trailers, or large RVs) just before the crest of the pass. Here, you'll find a sizable parking area (no charge), a restroom, and, at the highest point, a stone gazebo providing superb views into the Avra Valley west of Tucson; all are wheelchair-accessible. Highlights from the overlook include thick stands of saguaro, distant views of Old Tucson and the Arizona-Sonora Desert Museum, and romantic sunset vistas.

See the previous hike, Hike 24 (page 178), and Hike 25 (page 185) for other nearby attractions.

Directions

Drive west on Speedway Boulevard, one of Tucson's longest and most important east–west thoroughfares. (I-10 intersects Speedway at Exit 257.) Speedway becomes Gates Pass Road at Camino de Oeste, 4.8 miles west of I-10. If you're doing a car shuttle, turn left (south) on Camino de Oeste and drive 0.7 mile to the Camino de Oeste trailhead. *Note:* The last 0.2 mile is unpaved and has one-way sections, so use caution.

Back where Speedway becomes Gates Pass Road, continue west on Gates Pass. Drive over the pass (the overlook is about 2.5 miles beyond Camino de Oeste), and then carefully descend to the first parking lot on your left (south) for the David Yetman Trailhead, 3 miles along Gates Pass Road.

YOUNG SAGUAROS HANGING OUT WITH A VIEW OF GOLDEN GATE MOUNTAIN
(see Hike 28, page 202)

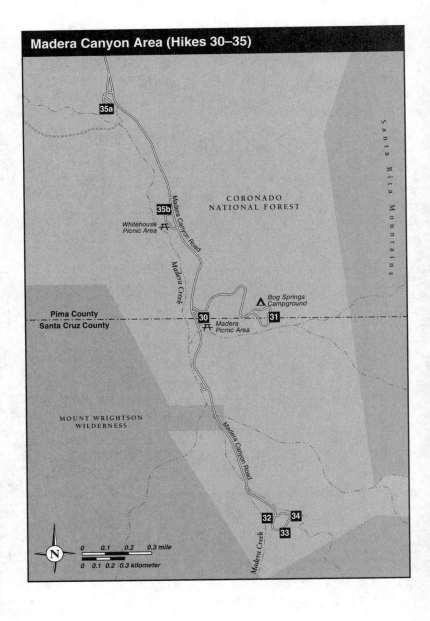

Madera Canyon Area (Hikes 30–35)

CORONADO
NATIONAL FOREST

Santa Rita Mountains

35a

Madera Canyon Road

35b

Whitehouse
Picnic Area

Madera Creek

Bog Springs
Campground

Pima County
Santa Cruz County

30   Madera
Picnic Area

31

MOUNT WRIGHTSON
WILDERNESS

Madera Canyon Road

32   34
33

Madera Creek

0   0.1   0.2   0.3 mile
0   0.1   0.2   0.3 kilometer

N

Madera Canyon Area

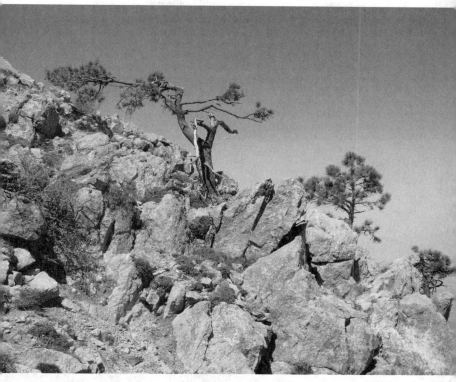

TWISTED PINE TREES NEAR THE SUMMIT OF MOUNT WRIGHTSON
(see Hike 33, page 236, and Hike 34, page 242)

30 Bog Springs–
Kent Spring Loop

SCENERY: ★ ★ ★ ★
TRAIL CONDITION: ★ ★ ★
CHILDREN: ★ ★ ★
DIFFICULTY: ★ ★ ★
SOLITUDE: ★ ★ ★ ★

TINY WATERFALLS TEASE THE HIKER ON KENT SPRING TRAIL.

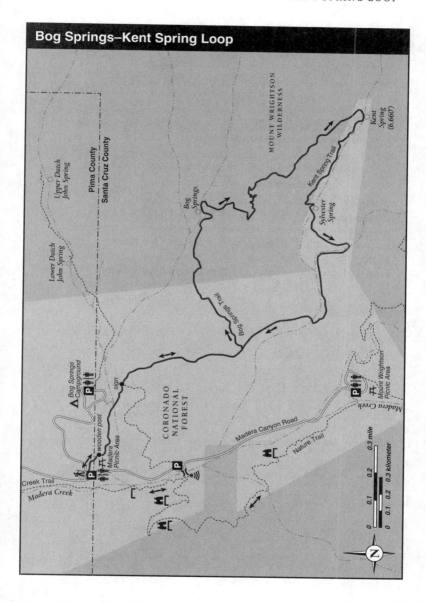

Bog Springs–Kent Spring Loop

MOUNT WRIGHTSON WILDERNESS

Kent Spring (6,660')

Bog Springs

Kent Spring Trail

Sylvester Spring

Upper Dutch John Spring

Pima County
Santa Cruz County

Lower Dutch John Spring

Bog Springs Trail

Bog Springs Campground

sign

CORONADO NATIONAL FOREST

wooden post

Madera Picnic Area

Mount Wrightson Picnic Area

Madera Creek

Madera Canyon Road

Nature Trail

Creek Trail

Madera Creek

0   0.1   0.2   0.3 mile

0   0.1   0.2   0.3 kilometer

N

GPS TRAILHEAD COORDINATES: N31° 43.606' W110° 52.810'

DISTANCE AND CONFIGURATION: 5.8-mile balloon

HIKING TIME: 3.75 hours

HIGHLIGHTS: Mountain and valley views, thick forest, three springs

ELEVATION: 4,840' at trailhead, 6,660' at Kent Spring

ACCESS: Open 24/7. Coronado Recreation Fee: $5/$10/$20 for day/week/year for up to 4 occupants of 1 car, available at picnic areas and at Santa Rita Lodge (see page 248); all National Park Service annual passes accepted.

MAPS: Green Trails *Maps 2962S–Santa Rita Mountains;* free trail map from Friends of Madera Canyon, available at trailheads and at the website below

FACILITIES: Restrooms, picnic tables, and water at the trailhead

WHEELCHAIR ACCESS: Restrooms and picnic tables at trailhead

COMMENTS: Leashed dogs and hikers only. There are three possible trailheads— I describe the route from Madera Picnic Area, with brief mentions of the trailheads at Bog Springs Campground and the Nature Trail and Amphitheater Parking Area.

CONTACTS: Friends of Madera Canyon, **friendsofmaderacanyon.org;** Coronado National Forest, Nogales Ranger District, 520-281-2296, **www.fs.usda.gov/coronado**

Overview

This loop takes you far from the desert and into thick and beautiful forests of sycamores, oaks, and pines. The Santa Rita Mountains are riddled with springs and streams that provide year-round moisture and support healthy woodlands. You pass three springs on this trail, at least two of which should have water year-round, but carry drinking water as the spring water is not clean. The streams are somewhat more intermittent, but they're gorgeous when they flow after snowmelt and after monsoon rains.

Route Details

The trailhead, with a map board, is on the east side of the Madera Picnic Area. Climb a narrow, rocky trail through mixed oak–juniper forest with agaves and yuccas scattered about. After 100 yards, join a wider trail and bear right (southeast); after another 100 yards, the trail forks left (east) again at a post with no sign on it. (Maybe this post will be removed or a sign will be restored—hang tough.) Here, go left and walk along the right side of a normally dry draw. The trail becomes rocky and somewhat faint but keeps heading east.

About 0.3 mile from the trailhead, the trail reaches a very rough dirt road. Here, if you take the road left (north), you'll drop down into the dry draw and hike up to Bog Springs Campground, 0.1 mile away. If you're camping, there is a signed trailhead with a map board for Bog Springs Trail, and you could begin from here.

If you wish to avoid the campground, just keep heading east on the dirt road. About 0.1 mile farther, you'll come to a metal sign on your left indicating that Bog and Kent Springs are ahead. The narrow, unsigned trail to the right (south) goes 0.6 mile to the Nature Trail and Amphitheater Parking Area on Madera Canyon Road—the third trailhead for this hike.

Beyond the metal sign, the going is much less complicated now that hikers from all three trailheads are on the same rocky road, originally built to reach Kent Spring but which hasn't seen a vehicle on it for years. The woodlands on either side of the road are thin, and deer roam the area—I saw a pair. Soon Mount Wrightson looms on the horizon to the southeast, and at some points it's dead ahead on the road.

About 0.5 mile beyond the last sign, you reach a signed fork where you can go either way on the ensuing 4-mile loop. Left goes to Bog Springs, right to Kent Spring. I prefer the clockwise loop: The section between Bog Springs and Kent Spring has the narrowest, steepest trail, and I like to climb it rather than descend it.

The left trail is a narrow one, and after a few hundred yards of climbing, views open to the left to the town of Green Valley to the northwest, 2,700 feet below and 12 miles away. Green areas around the town are pecan orchards, and the metallic-blue lake behind it is part of a mining operation. If conditions are clear, you might see Kitt and Baboquivari Peaks on the far distant horizon.

The trail enters thicker forest and, 0.8 mile from the beginning of the loop, a sign indicates Bog Springs to the left on a 0.1 mile dead-end trail that drops into and crosses a minor ravine before arriving

OAK WOODLANDS AND A YUCCA ALONG KENT SPRING ROAD

at the spring. The spring water is cached in a small, rectangular concrete basin surrounded by a lovely glade of pines and whitish Arizona sycamores, inviting further exploration. The water in the basin is greenish from fallen leaves and would require a good filter or several minutes of boiling to make it potable—typical for all the springs in these mountains. If you explore farther back, you'll find more water caches, which is why "Bog Springs" is plural. Once you're done, head back to the main trail.

Continue climbing briefly through tall, shady trees before emerging on a steep and exposed section, switchbacking up. You lose the shade but gain wonderful views of Mounts Wrightson and Hopkins. If you have a good eye (or binoculars), you can pick out Bog Springs Campground below. Eventually, the switchbacks end and the trail contours around to the south and then southeast, entering shade trees again. Kent Spring, reached 1.2 miles after Bog Springs, has a round concrete basin of dirty water. Just before it, a seasonal trickle is cleaner.

Our trail now turns hard right, drops west-northwest into a fern-filled little valley, and within a few yards becomes a steep, rough, and rather slippery shale-surfaced road. Watch your step! The seasonal stream may accompany you to your right if it was flowing just before Kent Spring. After a few hundred yards, the trail crosses the stream bed and becomes less steep. Trees bend over and provide a lovely shaded bower through which to continue your descent.

Soon you reach the third spring on the trail, Sylvester Spring, cached in two rectangular basins. The trail recrosses the stream bed and climbs briefly before dropping to another stream, this one flowing from left to right across your route. An unsigned trail climbs to your left if you want to explore the source of this stream. The Kent Spring Trail continues down, following the left bank of the stream through a gorgeous riparian area. At times, the stream disappears underground and pops up again a minute later.

About 0.1 mile before the Kent Spring Trail rejoins the Bog Springs Trail, a dirt road to your left (west) goes to the Kent Spring

Center, a 110-year-old house that's occasionally used for nature projects. Continue straight, but don't forget to look over your shoulder for views of Mount Wrightson lit by the afternoon sun. When you reach the sign for the Bog Springs Trail, continue north-northwest and then west for 0.9 mile, retracing your steps to the Madera Picnic Area.

Nearby Attractions

Bog Springs Campground (520-281-2296, **www.fs.usda.gov/coronado**) has 13 first-come, first-served sites, each featuring a picnic table and a fire ring with a barbecue grill. Drinking water and vault toilets are available; RV hookups aren't. Maximum vehicle length is limited to 22 feet. Fees are $10 per night. During weekends, especially in spring, summer, and fall, the campground can be full by lunchtime. The last time I camped here, I saw deer and wild turkeys near my tent in addition to the ever-present jays, woodpeckers, and squirrels. (There was also one small RV that insisted on running its loud generator at sunset until I had a quiet word with the owner.) Bearproof boxes are provided for your food; black bears may amble through every year or so.

Directions

From Tucson, follow the directions to the Visitor Information Station and Proctor Parking Area, as detailed in Hike 35 (page 249). Continue south on Madera Canyon Road for 1.1 miles to the Madera Picnic Area and trailhead. The road to Bog Springs Campground is on the left, just before the picnic area, and it's 0.5 mile to the campground. Signage is excellent.

Dutch John Spring Trail

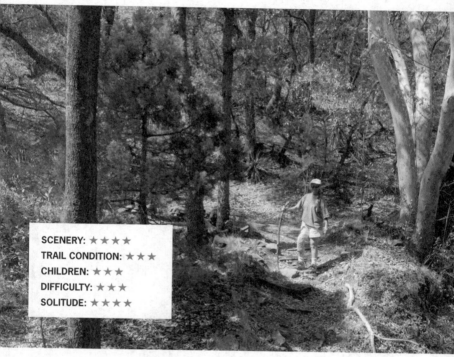

SCENERY: ★ ★ ★ ★
TRAIL CONDITION: ★ ★ ★
CHILDREN: ★ ★ ★
DIFFICULTY: ★ ★ ★
SOLITUDE: ★ ★ ★ ★

HIKING PAST THREE ARIZONA SYCAMORES ON THE DUTCH JOHN SPRING TRAIL

GPS TRAILHEAD COORDINATES: N31° 43.602' W110° 52.489'

DISTANCE & CONFIGURATION: 2.6-mile out-and-back

HIKING TIME: 2 hours

HIGHLIGHTS: Lovely woodlands, relative solitude on the upper trail

ELEVATION: 5,060' at trailhead, 6,000' at upper spring

ACCESS: Open 24/7. Coronado Recreation Fee: $5/$10/$20 for day/week/year for up to 4 occupants of 1 car, available at picnic areas and at Santa Rita Lodge (see page 248); all National Park Service annual passes accepted.

MAPS: Green Trails *Maps 2962S–Santa Rita Mountains;* free trail map from Friends of Madera Canyon, available at trailheads and at the website below

FACILITIES: Restrooms and water at the trailhead

WHEELCHAIR ACCESS: Restrooms at trailhead

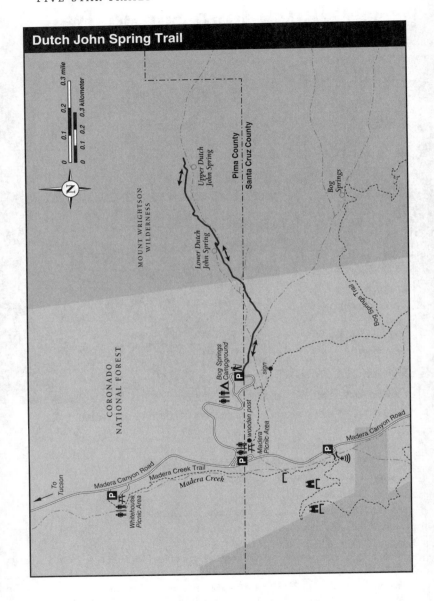

Dutch John Spring Trail

COMMENTS: Leashed dogs and hikers only. To make this hike almost a mile longer, begin from the Madera Picnic Area and follow the first two paragraphs of "Route Details" in the previous hike.

CONTACTS: Friends of Madera Canyon, **friendsofmaderacanyon.org**; Coronado National Forest, Nogales Ranger District, 520-281-2296, **www.fs.usda.gov/coronado**

Overview

This lovely woodland trail is just far enough away from Tucson that it gets few hikers. Most stop at the lower spring, and those continuing to the upper spring will either get lost or find solitude. (Audrey and I managed to do both!)

Route Details

The trailhead, which has an informative map board, is on the east side of Bog Springs Campground, behind the one restroom in this delightfully simple little campground. If you aren't camping here, four parking spaces by the trailhead are designated for hikers only. If you're hiking in from the Madera Canyon Picnic Area, when you get to the campground, just follow the road around to your right for a couple of hundred yards to the restroom and trailhead.

From the trailhead, you go east up a rocky trail between two campsites. After less than 0.1 mile you encounter a gate, which will let you through but keep horses out. Soon after, you'll cross a small ravine that looks like it should have water in it but rarely does. The trail, now pleasantly earthen instead of rocky, climbs gently through mixed woodland, soon reaching a four-strand wire fence on the right that marks one of the few areas of private land left in the canyon.

The plant life consists mainly of different kinds of oak trees, with agaves, yuccas, and the occasional lost-looking prickly pear cactus scattered through the woodland. Many of the oak species don't have the familiar deciduous, lobed leaves. Southern Arizona's plant life is enhanced by species that are mainly found in Mexico, such as Emory oaks, whose elongated, evergreen leaves can be smooth or toothed. These are shed but quickly replaced, and there are usually leaves on the ground year-round, not just in the fall. In several places along the trail, the oaks form a lovely bower overhead.

About 0.3 mile beyond the gate, the trail crosses the usually dry creek bed again and continues generally east or northeast. A quarter-mile farther brings you to a signed fork to the left indicating Dutch John Spring, just a few yards below you. A bathtub-sized metal trough here may be dry for much of the year. A half-dozen pale-barked Arizona sycamores surround the area, making for a very pretty glade.

Once you've finished exploring this area, which I call Lower Dutch John Spring, you can continue climbing on a narrow trail to the east-northeast, following the right side of the small ravine. Soon, you'll cross to the left side under three Arizona sycamores and come to a 12-foot-square dirt platform, shored up by a few rocks—I don't know what this is. About 0.3 mile from Lower Dutch John Spring, look for an unsigned fork that goes steeply to the right. (If you miss the turnoff and continue straight, staying on the left side of the creek bed, you'll be on a trail that swings north and peters out after a few hundred yards.)

The steep fork to the right soon becomes a gentle climb up the left side of another drainage. After a few hundred yards this becomes greener, and you may glimpse pools of water to your right, steeply but not far below. A mossy, glistening cliff on the far side appears to be the spring. If you cross the drainage to the right and start climbing a steep rock face, you've gone about 100 yards beyond the upper spring. There are no signs here.

So who was Dutch John? A locally respected historian, writer, and hiker spins a story about a murderous German gunslinger named John who worked in the Santa Rita Mountains in the 1920s, and whom locals thought might be Dutch. Perhaps they mistook his *Deutsch* for Dutch. (Truth be told, I found no history behind the name of this spring, so you're welcome to make up your own.)

Nearby Attractions

See the previous hike and Hike 34 (page 242) for details about camping or staying in Madera Canyon.

Directions

From Tucson, follow the directions to the Visitor Information Station and Proctor Parking Area, as detailed in Hike 35 (page 249). Continue south on Madera Canyon Road for 1.1 miles to a turnoff to the left for Bog Springs Campground, and drive 0.6 mile to the campground.

32

Nature Trail and Madera Creek Trail

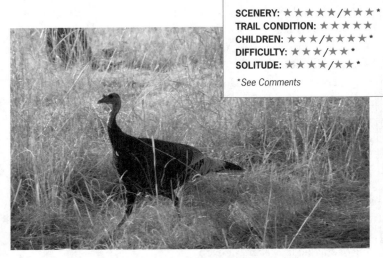

SCENERY: ★ ★ ★ ★ / ★ ★ ★ *
TRAIL CONDITION: ★ ★ ★ ★ ★
CHILDREN: ★ ★ ★ / ★ ★ ★ ★ *
DIFFICULTY: ★ ★ ★ / ★ ★ *
SOLITUDE: ★ ★ ★ ★ / ★ ★ *

*See Comments

WILD TURKEYS ARE COMMONLY HEARD AND SEEN IN MADERA CANYON.

GPS TRAILHEAD COORDINATES: N31° 42.792' W110° 52.498'

DISTANCE AND CONFIGURATION: 2.8-mile point-to-point with car shuttle, 5.6-mile out-and-back

HIKING TIME: 1.5 hours one-way

HIGHLIGHTS: Superb views of the mountain crest leading to Mount Wrightson; woodlands; riparian walk; bird-watching

ELEVATION: 5,420' at trailhead, 4,650' at trail's end

ACCESS: Open 24/7. Coronado Recreation Fee: $5/$10/$20 for day/week/year for up to 4 occupants of 1 car, available at picnic areas and at Santa Rita Lodge (see page 248); all National Park Service annual passes accepted.

MAPS: Green Trails *Maps 2962S–Santa Rita Mountains;* free trail map from Friends of Madera Canyon, available at trailheads and at the website below

FACILITIES: Restrooms, picnic tables, and water at the trailhead

WHEELCHAIR ACCESS: Restrooms and picnic tables at trailhead

COMMENTS: Leashed dogs and hikers only. The steeper Nature Trail (first set of star ratings) joins the easier Madera Creek Trail (second set of star ratings).

CONTACTS: Friends of Madera Canyon, **friendsofmaderacanyon.org;** Coronado National Forest, Nogales Ranger District, 520-281-2296, **www.fs.usda.gov/coronado**

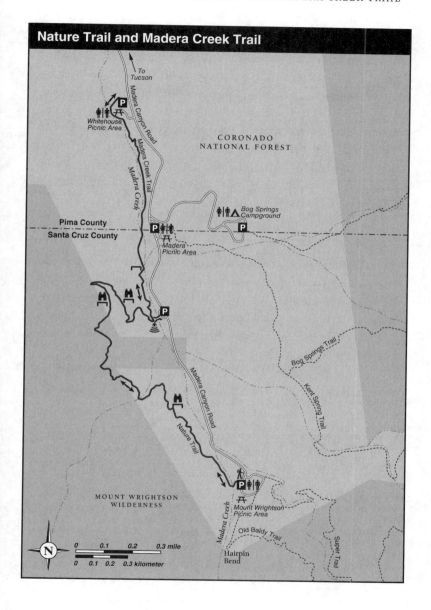

Nature Trail and Madera Creek Trail

To Tucson

Madera Canyon Road

Madera Creek Trail

Madera Creek

Whitehouse Picnic Area

CORONADO
NATIONAL FOREST

Bog Springs
Campground

Pima County
Santa Cruz County

Madera
Picnic Area

Bog Springs Trail

Kent Spring Trail

Madera Canyon Road

Nature Trail

Mount Wrightson
Picnic Area

MOUNT WRIGHTSON
WILDERNESS

Madera Creek

Old Baldy Trail

Super Trail

Hairpin
Bend

N

| 0 | 0.1 | 0.2 | 0.3 mile |

| 0 | 0.1 | 0.2 | 0.3 kilometer |

Overview

The upper section of the Nature Trail seems almost forgotten by hikers who are heading for the adjoining trailheads leading to the summit of Mount Wrightson, and there are relatively few people to be seen. Along the high trail, wooden benches are strategically placed for a relaxing rest and some of Madera Canyon's best views of Mount Wrightson. After undulating high above the valley, the route plunges down to Madera Creek, where a very popular trail parallels both the creek and the road but is just far enough away from the latter for birdsong to be heard.

Route Details

Begin from the west side of the extensive Mount Wrightson Picnic Area, at the far south terminus of the Madera Canyon Road. The trailhead is in the first parking lot on the right as you enter the picnic and parking area; you'll find a map board at the beginning of the trail. (Several other trails depart from this parking area, so make sure you're on the right one.)

From the trailhead, turn left (south), walk about 10 yards to cross a usually dry stream bed, and then switchback to the north, with the stream bed below to your right. After 100 yards, climb to your left away from the stream on a broken concrete trail. Soon you'll see the Chuparosa Inn across the stream to your right while you climb a little higher.

The trail quickly flattens and contours to the northwest, with Madera Creek dropping away below you. Although it seems fairly flat, the route actually undulates as it makes its way through mixed oak–juniper woodlands, with impressive yucca plants embellishing the trailside.

Past the first of several wooden benches, after about 0.6 mile, the Madera Creek Valley opens below. Occasional plaques at ground level identify trees growing alongside the trail. I like to stop at the second bench, a little over a mile from the trailhead, where there's a particularly impressive view of the Santa Ritas and a nearby plaque shows the peaks and landmarks neatly named for you, stretching from McCleary Peak to Mount Wrightson. The greener area surrounding Dutch John Spring is easy to make out and, with binoculars, Audrey and I were able to pick out our little blue-and-silver tent nestled in Bog Springs Campground. Fun stuff!

Shortly beyond the second bench, the trail hairpins and begins zigzagging down the hills toward the creek, with continuing great views. You pass a third bench. More signs interpret the geology and natural history of the canyon. Eventually, 1.8 miles from the trailhead, the route flattens and passes a small outdoor amphitheater used for ranger-led presentations and talks. Just before the amphitheater, to the right, a footbridge crosses Madera Creek and leads to the Nature Trail and Amphitheater Parking Area on Madera Canyon Road.

At this point, the Nature Trail becomes the Madera Creek Trail. With Santa Rita Lodge a short walk from the parking area, this segment of the trail is especially busy with walkers and bird-watchers. Water flows in this part of Madera Creek for much of the year, and frequent benches along the trail allow you to rest and enjoy the riparian scenery or listen to the sounds of birds and water. If you wish,

ARIZONA SYCAMORES AND HORSETAILS GROW ALONG MADERA CREEK.

you could return back to the trailhead the way you came, for a 3.6-mile out-and-back hike.

Continuing north from the amphitheater, the Madera Creek Trail starts by following the left bank and descending almost imperceptibly. Almost 0.5 mile from the amphitheater, the trail crosses the stream and passes through the west section of the Madera Picnic Area. (The east section, across the road, is the trailhead for the Bog Springs and Kent Spring Loop; see page 218.) After the picnic area, the trail passes through a very green, moist section with many horsetail plants. The creek is crossed a couple of times via wooden bridges before you arrive at the Whitehouse Picnic Area, 0.6 mile beyond the Madera Picnic Area. Here, one of the Wheelchair-Accessible Loops in Hike 35 begins (see page 249).

If you left a second vehicle here, you're finished; if not, it's back the way you came. Walking back along the road to the Mount Wrightson Picnic Area is a shorter return trip, but I don't recommend it because there's no sidewalk and the road is very narrow.

Nearby Attractions

See Hikes 30 and 34 (pages 218 and 242, respectively) for details about camping or staying in Madera Canyon.

Directions

From Tucson, follow the directions to the Whitehouse Picnic Area, as detailed in Hike 35 (page 249)—leave a car here if you're hiking one-way. To reach the Mount Wrightson Picnic Area and trailhead, continue south on Madera Canyon Road for 2.3 miles. Observe speed limits and drive carefully on this narrow road, which has one-lane bridges and pedestrian traffic.

Old Baldy Trail to Mount Wrightson

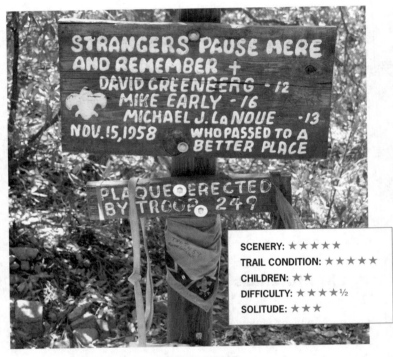

SCENERY: ★ ★ ★ ★ ★
TRAIL CONDITION: ★ ★ ★ ★ ★
CHILDREN: ★ ★
DIFFICULTY: ★ ★ ★ ★ ½
SOLITUDE: ★ ★ ★

THE BOY SCOUT MEMORIAL AT JOSEPHINE SADDLE

GPS TRAILHEAD COORDINATES: N31° 42.757' W110° 52.423'

DISTANCE AND CONFIGURATION: 10.8-mile out-and-back

HIKING TIME: 7 hours

HIGHLIGHTS: Summiting the highest peak in southern Arizona; beautiful forest and increasingly spectacular views

ELEVATION: 5,450' at trailhead, 9,453' at summit

ACCESS: Open 24/7. Coronado Recreation Fee: $5/$10/$20 for day/week/year for up to 4 occupants of 1 car, available at picnic areas and at Santa Rita Lodge (see page 248); all National Park Service annual passes accepted.

MAPS: Green Trails Maps 2962S–Santa Rita Mountains; free trail map from Friends of Madera Canyon, available at trailheads and at the website below

FACILITIES: Restrooms, picnic tables, and water at the trailhead

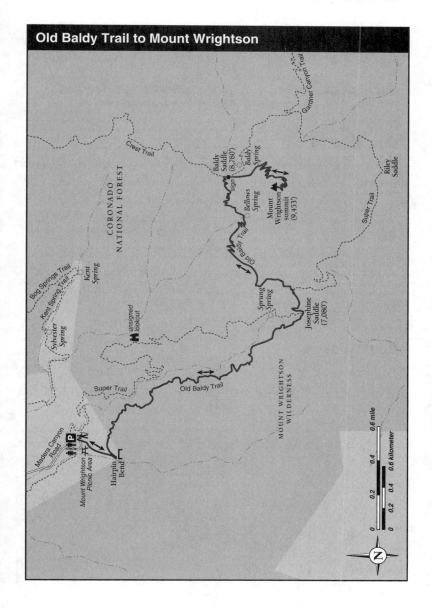

Old Baldy Trail to Mount Wrightson

Gardner Canyon Trail

Crest Trail

Baldy Saddle (8,780')

sign

Baldy Spring

Riley Saddle

CORONADO NATIONAL FOREST

Bellows Spring

Mount Wrightson summit (9,453')

Super Trail

Bog Springs Trail

Kent Spring Trail

Kent Spring

Sylvester Spring

Old Baldy Trail

unsigned lookout

Sprung Spring

Josephine Saddle (7,080')

Super Trail

Old Baldy Trail

MOUNT WRIGHTSON WILDERNESS

Madera Canyon Road

P

Mount Wrightson Picnic Area

Hairpin Bend

0   0.2   0.4   0.6 mile

0   0.2   0.4   0.6 kilometer

N

WHEELCHAIR ACCESS: Restrooms and picnic tables at trailhead

COMMENTS: Leashed dogs and hikers only. U.S. Forest Service signs, available maps, and other sources agree on a 10.8-mile out-and-back distance; my GPS tracked it at less than 10 miles.

CONTACTS: Friends of Madera Canyon, **friendsofmaderacanyon.org;** Coronado National Forest, Nogales Ranger District, 520-281-2296, **www.fs.usda.gov/coronado**

Overview

This is the oldest, shortest, and steepest route to ascend the 4,000 feet from the trailhead to summit. Desert dwellers can experience pleasing pine-forest smells, scenery, and shade while taking a break from the heat. The trail is very popular and occasionally becomes overrun with large hiking groups. With the exception of a few short, rocky sections near the summit, the trail is well maintained and makes the ascent surprisingly manageable, although the steep descent may take a toll on older knees. On a clear day, views stretch from northern Mexico to north of Tucson.

Route Details

Begin from the southeast end of the extensive Mount Wrightson Picnic Area, at the far south terminus of the Madera Canyon Road. You'll find an Old Baldy Trail map board at the beginning of this trail. (Several other trails depart from this picnic and parking area, so make sure you're on the right one.)

The first 0.25 mile follows a rough road (no vehicles) as it climbs southwest through thick forest to an intersection marked by two welded metal signs and a bench to rest on. One sign points the way southwest to Agua Caliente Saddle with the less-than-encouraging words "Very Steep Trail." Although this isn't our route, it is noteworthy that the first section of this trail, before it gets very steep, is popular with birders looking for the elegant trogon, a parrot-like bird from Central America. The trogon's northernmost limit is a few canyons in southeastern Arizona and southwestern New Mexico, with Madera Canyon being a hot spot; this trail section is among the best places to see trogons. The birds nest here from April to August and head as far south as Costa Rica in the fall and winter. The male's striking red, white, and green plumage is unmistakable, and it is only one of many species that make a bird-watching expedition to the canyon a memorable event.

Another sign at this intersection points out the Old Baldy Trail, which makes a hairpin bend to the left and climbs steadily but gently, swinging around from northeast to southeast and following the right (west) side of the Madera Creek valley. Once, when Audrey and I hiked up this trail, we saw a black bear browsing in that valley, about a hundred feet below. We quietly kept climbing and it ignored us, but we finished that day with a great story to tell.

There are no especially difficult or remarkable stretches on the 2.5-mile climb from the trailhead to Josephine Saddle, at 7,080 feet. The lower parts traverse mixed deciduous oak forests with the occasional conifer, but when you reach Josephine Saddle evergreens begin to dominate. The trail, climbing steadily with occasional flattish sections, is mainly comfortably earthen with a few roots and rocks. You'll glimpse Mount Wrightson to the southeast and east, but mostly you'll enjoy forest hiking.

At Josephine Saddle stands a rustic memorial cross to three teenage boys—members of Boy Scout Troop 249, who were caught by an unseasonably early winter storm on November 15, 1958, and died of hypothermia. Passing hikers and Scouts leave tributes, and the memorial looks slightly different from month to month.

Six trails meet at Josephine Saddle, and there are several signs to sort them out. Old Baldy Trail and the Super Trail (see next hike) follow the same route for a short section heading left (northeast) on the trail signed for Mount Wrightson. About 40 yards beyond the Boy Scout cross, the trail forks, and you go left to climb a couple of switchbacks. There are good views of the observatories on Mount Hopkins just south of west and the distinctively triangular peak of Pete Mountain to the northwest. About 0.2 mile above Josephine Saddle, the Super Trail goes off to the right and Old Baldy Trail goes more or less straight east and then swings north. It's 4.2 miles to Mount Wrightson via the Super Trail or 2.7 miles via Old Baldy.

As the trail climbs, views open to the northwest of the town of Green Valley, with a metallic-blue lake, the result of a mining operation, behind it. Soon after, the trail becomes rockier, the gradient increases, and you begin switchbacking through thinning trees, some of which show evidence of past forest fires. Just over a mile beyond the intersection with the Super Trail, the trail flattens and you'll pass Bellows Spring to your right, at 8,170 feet elevation. A small, verdant cliff above the trail shines with water seeps, which are collected in a little stone and concrete basin right by the trail. This water should be filtered or boiled before drinking.

After Bellows Spring, the trail continues switchbacking through a mixture of pine trees and bare, colorful rock cliffs, some of which are rusty with iron ore. Another 0.7 mile of climbing takes you to the 8,780-foot Baldy Saddle, where expansive views open of distant mountain ranges to the east and Gardner Canyon below. Back to the west-southwest, you're now looking down on observatory-topped Mount Hopkins; to the south, the bald cliffs of Mount Wrightson appear an impossibly steep 0.9 mile away. You can see how the mountain got its original name of Old Baldy.

About 100 yards south of Baldy Saddle, a metal sign points to Gardner Canyon down to the left (southeast)—this is the descent via the Super Trail. Both the Super and Old Baldy Trails now follow the same route to the summit, climbing gently south and contouring around the northeast side of the mountain through pine forest. The final push to the top begins suddenly, with a long series of rocky switchbacks that end equally suddenly at the summit.

There used to be a fire lookout perched on the top, but only foundations remain, accompanied by a couple of waterproof ammo boxes that hold trail registers. An informative plaque tells the history of the lookout. The views can be awesome on a clear day. Unfortunately, there is an increasing number of hazy days when the horizon is totally obscured by smog or smoke—hopefully, you'll be here on a pristine day with jaw-dropping vistas.

Nearby Attractions

See the next hike and Hike 30 (page 218) for details about camping or staying in Madera Canyon.

Directions

From Tucson, follow the directions to the Visitor Information Station and Proctor Parking Area, as detailed in Hike 35 (page 249). Continue south on Madera Canyon Road for 2.3 miles to the Mount Wrightson Picnic Area and trailhead. Observe speed limits and drive carefully on this narrow road, which has one-lane bridges and pedestrian traffic.

34 Super Trail to Mount Wrightson

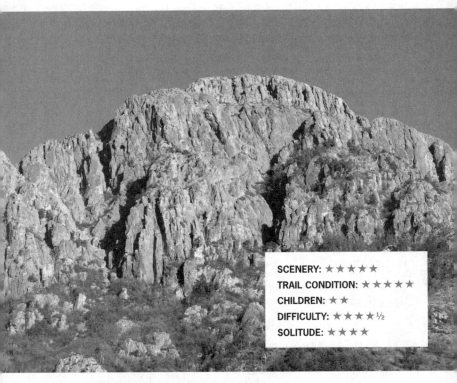

SCENERY: ★ ★ ★ ★ ★
TRAIL CONDITION: ★ ★ ★ ★ ★
CHILDREN: ★ ★
DIFFICULTY: ★ ★ ★ ★ ½
SOLITUDE: ★ ★ ★ ★

MOUNT WRIGHTSON IN THE AFTERNOON SUN

GPS TRAILHEAD COORDINATES: N31° 42.811' W110° 52.392'

DISTANCE AND CONFIGURATION: 16.2-mile out-and-back

HIKING TIME: 10.5 hours

HIGHLIGHTS: Beautiful forests; great views of the high crest leading north of Mount Wrightson; summit of southern Arizona's highest peak

ELEVATION: 5,425' at trailhead, 9,453' at summit

ACCESS: Open 24/7. Coronado Recreation Fee: $5/$10/$20 for day/week/year for up to 4 occupants of 1 car, available at picnic areas and at Santa Rita Lodge (see Nearby Attractions); all National Park Service annual passes accepted.

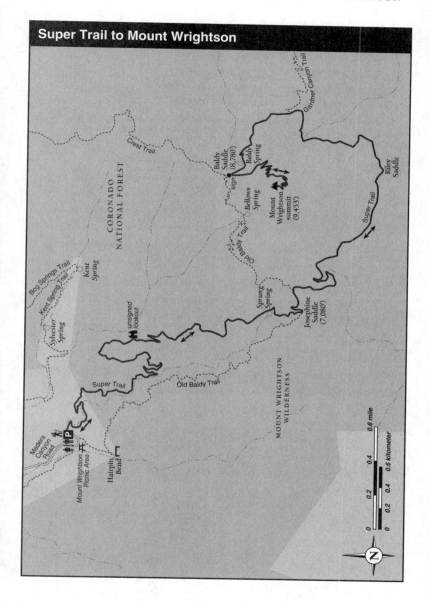

Super Trail to Mount Wrightson

MAPS: Green Trails *Maps 2962S–Santa Rita Mountains;* free trail map from Friends of Madera Canyon, available at trailheads and at the website below

FACILITIES: Restrooms, picnic tables, and water at the trailhead

WHEELCHAIR ACCESS: Restrooms and picnic tables at trailhead

COMMENTS: Leashed dogs and hikers only. U.S. Forest Service signs, available maps, and other sources agree on a 16.2-mile out-and-back distance; my GPS tracked it at 15.4 miles.

CONTACTS: Friends of Madera Canyon, **friendsofmaderacanyon.org;** Coronado National Forest, Nogales Ranger District, 520-281-2296, **www.fs.usda.gov/coronado**

Overview

This is a newer, longer, and more gradual route to ascend the 4,000 feet from the trailhead to Mount Wrightson's summit. But what it gains in being less steep is lost in distance—it's not an easier trail. The lower sections have some attractive riparian areas, and pine forests provide shaded hiking up to Josephine Saddle, where the Super Trail coincides briefly with the Old Baldy Trail. Then the Super Trail almost circumnavigates the mountain as far as Baldy Saddle, where it again overlaps with Old Baldy for the last 0.9 mile to the summit, including the steepest section of this route.

Using the intersection with Old Baldy at Josephine Saddle, hikers can create a number of loops or a figure-eight, so that several ascents can be made without repeating exactly the same path.

Route Details

Begin from the northeast end of the extensive Mount Wrightson Picnic Area, at the far south terminus of the Madera Canyon Road. When you enter the picnic and parking area, drive almost all the way around it to a restroom at the northeast corner. The trail begins behind this restroom; you'll find a Super Trail map board at the trailhead. (Several other trails depart from this parking area, so make sure you're on the right one.)

Head east from the parking lot and soon follow the right bank of Madera Creek about 0.3 mile. Here, the trail crosses the creek at a point marked by three majestic Arizona sycamores, then continues up the other side heading west briefly. (There probably won't be any water in the creek from late spring until the monsoon season.) The trail switchbacks up the far side of the creek in long, gentle ascents, which change direction to all points of the compass. Deciduous forest begins to give way to coniferous as you climb, and there are frequent glimpses of Mount Wrightson to the southeast and Mount Hopkins to the southwest.

About 2 miles from the trailhead, you'll have climbed about 1,000 feet. Views open to the left of the trail and between the trees of the main crest of the Santa Ritas, including the three highest peaks in these mountains. Mount Wrightson is the farthest southeast. Mount Ian (simply marked as 9,146 on most maps) is to the east, and to the northeast an unnamed peak (marked 8,853) is the third highest. Somebody needs to come up with a fitting name for this significant summit! If you're trying to get the best views between the trees, keep your eyes open for a flat, unsigned lookout on the left side of the trail.

The next landmark, about 1.5 miles farther, is the delightfully named Sprung Spring, which fills a round metal basin on the right side of the trail. The water looks clear but should always be purified. You're now just 0.25 mile from Josephine Saddle, which is 3.7 miles from the trailhead. The Super Trail enters the saddle opposite the Boy Scout memorial cross (see page 239) and turns left, following the same route as the Old Baldy Trail for 0.2 mile. A metal sign clearly marks where the Super Trail turns off Old Baldy to the right (south). From this fork, it's 4.2 miles to Mount Wrightson via the Super Trail or 2.7 miles via Old Baldy.

The next section swings around the southwestern side of Mount Wrightson, climbing occasional switchbacks and yielding excellent views of Mount Hopkins to the west. You'll encounter a few brief loose sections as the trail crosses small, rocky landslides, but none are a problem. About 1.4 miles of hiking from the previous trail fork will bring you to the 8,000-foot contour and Riley Saddle, on the south side of the mountain. A signed but poorly maintained trail from here goes south toward Josephine Peak, which has tree trunks scattered on it like matchsticks. No one seems to know who Josephine was, but she has the fifth highest peak in the Santa Ritas, a saddle, and a canyon named after her.

SONORAN MOUNTAIN KING SNAKE

The Super Trail continues swinging around the south and southeast sides of Mount Wrightson. The next section is notable for the thick, scratchy graythorn bushes encroaching on the trail—you might want to wear long pants. As you climb around to the east side, you'll see increasingly burned-out areas, remnants of the Florida Fire of 2005. The signed junction with the Gardner Trail is 1.1 miles beyond Riley Saddle. By this point you're surrounded by a surreal landscape of burned, dead trees.

From this junction it's a 0.8-mile climb to Baldy Saddle. Much of this section has fallen trees across it, so your ascent is slowed as you make your way around or over the obstacles. About 0.15 mile before the saddle, you'll pass Baldy Spring, which used to be a reliable source of water; since the fire, however, the bathtub-sized green metal basin used for catchment is often dry.

The Super Trail terminates at Baldy Saddle. The familiar metal sign indicates that Mount Wrightson is 0.9 mile to your left, and you follow the same route as Old Baldy Trail to the summit. To reach the heart of Baldy Saddle, turn right and walk 100 yards.

The mountain used to be called Old Baldy because of its rocky, treeless summit but is now named after William Wrightson, a mining surveyor who was killed by Apaches in 1865. Nearby Mount Hopkins is named after Gilbert Hopkins, a mining engineer who was killed in the same attack.

A remarkable natural feature of the summit is ladybugs. Most of the year you won't see any, but in early summer (around June) these familiar red insects with the black spots swarm the summit by the thousands to breed. Don't worry—they don't bite!

Nearby Attractions

While it's possible to climb Mount Wrightson with a dawn departure from Tucson, some hikers prefer to stay nearer the mountain. You can camp (see Hike 30, page 218) or stay in one of three rustic lodges in Madera Canyon. These offer standard rooms with kitchenettes, and guests bring their own food. None of them are luxurious, but they do offer a pleasant getaway from the desert. The nearest stores and restaurants are in Green Valley, 15 miles away. During the spring and early-summer birding seasons, reservations are advised.

The largest and best-known lodge is **Santa Rita Lodge** (520-625-8746, **santaritalodge.com**), with about a dozen rooms and cabins, mostly in the $110–$130 range at press time. A small store sells souvenirs, maps, books, drinks, and snacks, and a bird-watching station is open to the public. The tiny **Madera Kubo** (520-625-9208, **maderakubo .com**) has four Hobbit-sized cabins (two with spiral stairways) and a souvenir shop. Rates are $110 for one night or $95 for multiple nights. The **Chuparosa Inn** (520-393-7370, **chuparosainn.com**) has four nice rooms in the $150–$200 range and serves a Continental breakfast.

Directions

From Tucson, follow the directions to the Visitor Information Station and Proctor Parking Area, as detailed in the next hike. Continue south on Madera Canyon Road for 2.3 miles to the Mount Wrightson Picnic Area and trailhead. Observe speed limits and drive carefully on this narrow road, which has one-lane bridges and pedestrian traffic. Drive all the way around the large parking area to the trailhead.

Madera Canyon:
Wheelchair-Accessible Loops

OCOTILLOS AND ELEPHANT HEAD SEEN FROM PROCTOR LOOP TRAIL

GPS TRAILHEAD COORDINATES: Proctor Parking Area Trailhead, N31° 44.467' W110° 53.215'; Whitehouse Picnic Area Trailhead, N31° 44.026' W110° 52.950'

DISTANCE AND CONFIGURATION: 0.8-mile loop from Proctor Parking Area Trailhead; 0.5-mile loop from Whitehouse Picnic Area Trailhead; 1.5-mile figure-eight

HIKING TIME: As long as you want

HIGHLIGHTS: Wheelchair access, nice mix of mountain views, high desert woodlands, and historical markers

ELEVATION: 4,450' at Proctor Parking Area, 4,650' at Whitehouse Picnic Area; no significant rise

ACCESS: Open 24/7. Coronado Recreation Fee: $5/$10/$20 for day/week/year for up to 4 occupants of 1 car, available at picnic areas and at Santa Rita Lodge (see page 248); all National Park Service annual passes accepted.

MAPS: Green Trails *Maps 2962S–Santa Rita Mountains;* free trail map from Friends of Madera Canyon, available at trailheads and at the website below

FACILITIES: Restrooms and water at both trailheads

WHEELCHAIR ACCESS: Restrooms, picnic tables, and both loop trails, but not the short connector trail

Madera Canyon: Wheelchair-Accessible Loops

Madera Canyon Road

Proctor Parking Area

Madera Creek

White House ruin

Proctor Road

CORONADO NATIONAL FOREST

Madera Creek

Madera Canyon Road

Loop Trail

grave of unknown pioneer

Whitehouse Picnic Area

Madera Creek Trail

N

0   200   400   600 feet
0   50   100   150 meters

COMMENTS: Leashed dogs and hikers only. The two paved loops are at least 42 inches wide.

CONTACTS: Friends of Madera Canyon, **friendsofmaderacanyon.org**; Coronado National Forest, Nogales Ranger District, 520-281-2296, **www.fs.usda.gov/coronado**

Overview

These two loops are lovely. Folks in wheelchairs will definitely get a real outdoors experience with fine mountain views, bird-filled woodlands, and historical sites. The trails are also recommended for slower hikers who use a cane or don't want to climb. Bird-watchers and visitors with limited time enjoy the easy hike and the informative signs along the trails. The Proctor Trailhead has an informative shaded ramada detailing the history and natural history of Madera Canyon, along with a visitor center that's open most weekends. The Whitehouse Trailhead has a picnic area.

Route Details

I describe the Proctor Loop first. Read further for the shorter Whitehouse Loop.

From the Proctor Parking Area, the paved trail goes south. After 100 yards, a plaque on the right side of the trail identifies the mountains to the west of you, visible on a clear day. A couple of hundred yards farther, a 20-yard-long side trail takes you to a huge Arizona sycamore that provides shade over a bench.

Back on the main trail, you'll cross the unpaved Proctor Road (a brief but not insurmountable inconvenience to wheelchair users), soon followed by a signed left turn to the White House ruin, easily reached on a very short paved trail. A century ago, these adobe walls were whitewashed, and the house was a major landmark—indeed, the original name of the canyon was White House Canyon. Today, only a single wall remains.

According to the book *A History of Madera Canyon*, published by the Friends of Madera Canyon, the White House was built around

1880 and had several owners and inhabitants until 1940. The last full-time inhabitants were Alcaro Morales (61), who moved here in 1911 with his bride, Benita (27). He helped his wife give birth to four children, but sadly, she and their fifth child died in childbirth in 1921. The family continued to live here, supporting themselves by selling vegetables, cheese, pine nuts, and mescal, until Alcaro's death in 1940.

THE SHADED LOWER PROCTOR LOOP TRAIL

Just beyond the White House trail, the Bat House exhibit is on your left. Four bat houses have been placed on tall poles, and a well-illustrated plaque explains that 17 of the 45 bat species found in the United States and Canada have been recorded in Madera Canyon. The best time to see bats is at sunset, when they become active, especially in the spring and summer. Please don't disturb the bats, and stay on the trail.

A few yards past the bat houses and 0.24 mile from the trailhead, the trail forks into a 0.35-mile loop that you can take either way. Going right, you'll quickly come to a wooden bridge crossing Madera Creek, which will be dry in late spring and summer. About halfway around the paved loop, you'll reach the signed intersection with the unpaved Upper Loop Trail. This 0.2-mile-long trail links with the Whitehouse Loop, and hikers can use it to make a figure-eight excursion. Wheelchair users will continue around the paved loop, crossing another wooden bridge over Madera Creek and returning to the Proctor Parking Area.

It's a 0.7-mile drive from the Proctor Parking Area to the Whitehouse Picnic Area, where the second paved, wheelchair-accessible loop begins. Heading right from the trailhead, you'll pass a short, paved side trail to the grave of an unknown pioneer; a short way farther are three more bat houses with an accompanying informative plaque. The trail is surrounded by the pine–oak woodlands typical of this elevation.

Roughly halfway around the paved loop, the signed, unpaved Lower Loop Trail takes hikers 0.2 mile to the Proctor Loop for a figure-eight. Wheelchair users continue around the paved loop to a fork that gives access to a Madera Creek overlook, to the right via a 0.1-mile paved trail. The main loop trail passes a few remnants of a 1930s Depression-era Civilian Conservation Corps camp, where hundreds of young men were housed and employed by the national forest. The end of the loop coincides with the last few yards of the Madera Creek Trail.

Nearby Attractions

See the previous hike and Hike 30 (page 218) for information about camping and lodging in Madera Canyon.

Directions

From Tucson, take I-19 south. This short freeway begins in south Tucson at I-10 and continues to the U.S.–Mexico border at Nogales, with distances marked in kilometers. From the I-10 exit, it's 38 kilometers (about 24 miles) along I-19 to Exit 63/Continental Road. Take Continental Road east for 1.2 miles to White House Canyon Road. Here, turn right and drive 7.1 miles to Madera Canyon Road, where you turn right again and drive 3.5 miles to the Visitor Information Station (open most weekends, 10 a.m.–2 p.m.) and the adjoining Proctor Parking Area.

The Proctor Parking Area is the trailhead of the first wheelchair-accessible loop. To get to the second loop, turn right out of the Proctor Parking Area and drive 0.7 mile south to the Whitehouse Picnic Area.

Appendix A:
Outdoor Retailers

Perhaps because the weather here is so ideal and folks don't need down jackets, four-season tents, and snowshoes, Tucson has surprisingly few outdoors stores that sell high-quality hiking equipment. Here are some that do.

MILLER'S SURPLUS millerssurplus.com
Old-fashioned army surplus—you never know what they might have!

406 N. 6th Ave.
Tucson, AZ 85705
520-441-1099

1537 S. Craycroft Rd.
Tucson, AZ 85711
520-790-8700

REI rei.com
160 W. Wetmore Rd.
Tucson, AZ 85705
520-887-1938

SUMMIT HUT summithut.com
In business since 1969, this is Tucson's oldest—and only—independent outdoors retailer, and warmly recommended.

5045 E. Speedway Blvd.
Tucson, AZ 85712
520-325-1554

7745 N. Oracle Rd.
Tucson, AZ 85704
520-888-1000

WESTERN NATIONAL PARKS ASSOCIATION (WNPA) wnpa.org
The hiking gear is limited, but the WNPA sells Tucson's widest selection of books and gifts for the outdoors enthusiast.

12880 N. Vistoso Village Dr.
Tucson, AZ 85755
520-622-6014

Appendix B: Map Resources

U.S. Geological Survey (USGS) topo maps are accurate but often lack trails. I like **Green Trails** maps—three cover the Santa Catalina Mountains, Santa Rita Mountains, and Saguaro area—and **National Geographic**'s Saguaro National Park maps, which are based on USGS topographical information and show hiking trails as well. The **U.S. Forest Service** map of Pusch Ridge is also useful.

The stores in Appendix A and the visitor centers listed for hikes in Saguaro National Park, Sabino Canyon, and Catalina State Park sell all of the above; you can also buy them at the sources below.

GREEN TRAILS MAPS   greentrailsmaps.com

NATIONAL GEOGRAPHIC MAPS   maps.nationalgeographic.com/maps

TUCSON'S MAP AND FLAG CENTER   mapsmithus.com
Carries every topo map of Arizona, and maps of everywhere else.
    3239 N. 1st Ave.
    Tucson, AZ 85719
    520-887-4234

U.S. GEOLOGICAL SURVEY   nationalmap.gov, usgs.gov

Appendix C: Hiking Clubs

Local hiking groups meet online as well as on the trail.

SIERRA CLUB–GRAND CANYON CHAPTER, RINCON GROUP
arizona.sierraclub.org/rincon
    738 N. 5th Ave., Ste. 214
    Tucson, AZ 85705
    520-620-6401

SOUTHERN ARIZONA HIKING CLUB   ahcinfo.org
    P.O. Box 32257
    Tucson, AZ 85715

THE RAMBLERS   clubs.arizona.edu/~ramblers
One of the University of Arizona's oldest student organizations;
open to all Tucson hikers.

THE TUCSON HIKING MEETUP GROUP   meetup.com/tucsonhiking

Index

About the Author

Photo: Todd Jones

ROB RACHOWIECKI was raised in London and climbed his first mountain by accident, while on a school biology field course in Scotland. After a day of dissecting newts, he walked to the top of a windswept hill behind the outdoor studies center, looked around at miles of startling wilderness, and had an "I'm the king of the world!" revelation.

Rob crossed the pond in 1974, planning on traveling around the world but ending up living and traveling throughout the Americas, from Alaska to Argentina. He has authored hiking and climbing guides to Central America and the Central Andes, as well as travel guides to Peru, Ecuador, Costa Rica, and the American Southwest for publishers ranging from Lonely Planet to National Geographic. He has been an active member of the Society of American Travel Writers since 1997.

From 1983 to 2008, Rob worked as an adventure-travel guide, leading treks in the Andes and adventures on the Amazon. Since 1990 he has lived in Tucson, where he earned a master's degree at the University of Arizona and where he enjoys the area's varied ethnic restaurants, theatres, and outdoor music festivals. He is often found hiking the many desert, canyon, and mountain trails surrounding Tucson, following the seasonal changes and usually doing a spot of bird-watching, as Brits are wont to do.

Since 2006, Rob has worked a day job as a respiratory therapist at a superb rural community hospital in Benson, near Tucson. He collects armadillos—sculptures, not live ones!—and owns 19 at last count. He wears size-13 hiking boots and does not own a suit. He plays a decent game of Scrabble but is a weak (though enthusiastic) chess player. However, he finds playing 20 Questions easier on the trail than trying to balance all those little pieces.

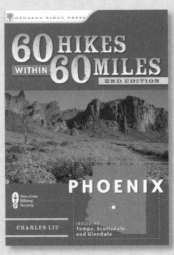